International Perspectives on Social Policy, Administration, and Practice

Series Editor

Sheying Chen
Pace University, New York, NY, USA

Jason L. Powell
University of Lancashire, Preston, Lancashire, United Kingdom

The Springer series International Perspectives on Social Policy, Administration and Practice puts the spotlight on international and comparative studies of social policy, administration, and practice with an up-to-date assessment of their character and development. In particular, the series seeks to examine the underlying assumptions of the practice of helping professions, nonprofit organization and management, and public policy and how processes of both nation-state and globalization are affecting them. The series also includes specific country case studies, with valuable comparative analysis across Asian, African, Latin American, and Western welfare states. The series International Perspectives on Social Policy, Administration and Practice commissions approximately six books per year, focusing on international perspectives on social policy, administration, and practice, especially an East-West connection. It assembles an impressive set of researchers from diverse countries illuminating a rich, deep, and broad understanding of the implications of comparative accounts on international social policy, administration, and practice.

More information about this series at http://www.springer.com/series/7

Steven L. Arxer • John W. Murphy
Editors

Dimensions of Community-Based Projects in Health Care

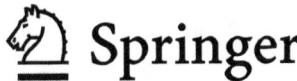
Springer

Editors
Steven L. Arxer
Department of Sociology & Psychology
University of North Texas at Dallas
Dallas, TX, USA

John W. Murphy
Department of Sociology
University of Miami
Coral Gables, FL, USA

International Perspectives on Social Policy, Administration, and Practice
ISBN 978-3-319-61556-1   ISBN 978-3-319-61557-8 (eBook)
DOI 10.1007/978-3-319-61557-8

Library of Congress Control Number: 2017953040

© Springer International Publishing AG 2018
This work is subject to copyright. All rights are reserved by the Publisher, whether the whole or part of the material is concerned, specifically the rights of translation, reprinting, reuse of illustrations, recitation, broadcasting, reproduction on microfilms or in any other physical way, and transmission or information storage and retrieval, electronic adaptation, computer software, or by similar or dissimilar methodology now known or hereafter developed.
The use of general descriptive names, registered names, trademarks, service marks, etc. in this publication does not imply, even in the absence of a specific statement, that such names are exempt from the relevant protective laws and regulations and therefore free for general use.
The publisher, the authors and the editors are safe to assume that the advice and information in this book are believed to be true and accurate at the date of publication. Neither the publisher nor the authors or the editors give a warranty, express or implied, with respect to the material contained herein or for any errors or omissions that may have been made. The publisher remains neutral with regard to jurisdictional claims in published maps and institutional affiliations.

Printed on acid-free paper

This Springer imprint is published by Springer Nature
The registered company is Springer International Publishing AG
The registered company address is: Gewerbestrasse 11, 6330 Cham, Switzerland

Preface

Community-based approaches are popular today in the area of social services, especially as proposals to decentralize health care gain traction. Part of the appeal comes from the recognition that traditional health care management has led to higher costs and to services unresponsive to the population. Many communities are still caught in the effects of the Great Recession and are seeking control over their lives. A basic assumption of this change to community-based health care delivery is that health services will be more attuned to the needs of community members and sustainable over time.

A central theme of this book is that a shift in social philosophy is needed for a community-based approach to health care. Most important to recognize is that the usual way of imagining community-based interventions may be insufficient. For although conventional health projects may at times be linked to communities, these ties may fail to be sensitive to the participatory nature specified by community-based theory. As a result, the practices and frameworks developed from these efforts become divorced from critical reflection and widespread dialogue.

In this book, readers are encouraged to rethink the basic but important aspects of community-based theory—namely, that community should not be simplified within community-based programs. In other words, the goal is not merely to be more efficient in social service delivery. While this outcome is expected, community-based practitioners are primarily interested in engaging communities in a manner that promotes participation by the citizenry. Simply stated, the open and democratic character of this philosophy represents what is "new" about community-based theory and related health projects.

However, a community-based approach is also more than a philosophy. Included are practical considerations, such as new methodologies, leadership styles, and organizational management strategies. In general, the language and planning of health care must be rethought. Examples are provided in this book that illustrate the various dimensions of a community-based strategy. Central to these efforts is that a "participatory culture" is promoted, whereby community members begin to direct—and, perhaps, even begin to control—intervention programs. The hope is that this book helps both academics and practitioners to establish a link between novel philosophical insights and the practice of developing community-based projects. In this way, community-based interventions can offer an alternative mode of service delivery that is responsive to communities and contributes to the improvement of health outcomes.

Dallas, TX, USA Steven L. Arxer
Coral Gables, FL, USA John W. Murphy

Contents

1. **Introduction**.. 1
   Steven L. Arxer and John W. Murphy

2. **Narrative Medicine in the Context of Community-Based Practice** ... 15
   John W. Murphy

3. **Qualitative and Participatory Action Research** 25
   Steven L. Arxer, Maria del Puy Ciriza, and Marco Shappeck

4. **Health Committees as a Community-Based Strategy** 37
   Berkeley Franz, Chantelle Shaw, and Keilah Ketron

5. **Dialogue, World Entry, and Community-Based Intervention** 55
   Jung Min Choi

6. **Politics of Knowledge in Community-Based Work** 67
   Karie Jo Peralta

7. **Community Mapping Tells an Important Story** 79
   Karen A. Callaghan

8. **Training Physicians with Communities** 93
   David Laubli, Daniel Skinner, and Kyle Rosenberger

9. **A Community-Based Approach to Primary Health Care**........... 105
   Khary K. Rigg, Doug Engelman, and Jesús Ramirez

10. **Conclusion: Reimagining Community Planning in Health Care**..... 119
    Steven L. Arxer and John W. Murphy

Index... 129

Contributors

Steven L. Arxer is associate professor at the University of North Texas at Dallas in the Department of Sociology and Psychology. He specializes in qualitative research on minority populations, with a focus on intersectionality, aging, and globalization. He is coauthor of *Aging in a Second Language*.

Karen A. Callaghan is professor of sociology and dean of the College of Arts and Sciences at Barry University, Miami Shores, Florida. She received her Ph.D. from Ohio State University. Her present interests include community-based research and organizing, social inequalities, and sociology of education.

Jung Min Choi is associate professor of sociology at San Diego State University. He received his Ph.D. from York University in Toronto, Canada. He has published numerous books, book chapters, and articles in the areas of postmodern/poststructural theory, multicultural identity, critical pedagogy, and narrative health.

Maria del Puy Ciriza is assistant professor of Spanish at Texas Christian University, Fort Worth. She received her Ph.D. from the University of Illinois. Her current research focuses on sociolinguistics concretely on issues of language and identity.

Doug Engelman is a doctoral student in sociology at the University of South Florida, Tampa, where his concentrations are in health and illness and the sociology of education. He received his M.A. in sociology at Northern Illinois University.

Berkeley Franz is an assistant professor of social medicine at Ohio University's Heritage College of Osteopathic Medicine. She received her Ph.D. in sociology from the University of Miami. Her research and teaching interests include community-based health interventions, health policy, and the sociology of religion.

Keilah Ketron is a second year medical student at Ohio University's Heritage College of Osteopathic Medicine. She is in the Rural and Urban Scholars Pathway Program with the intention of practicing family medicine in an underserved community. She has a B.A. in biology from Cedarville University.

David Laubli, BS is a third year medical student at Ohio University's Heritage College of Osteopathic Medicine. His interests include simulation in medical education and value-based medicine.

John W. Murphy has a Ph.D. in sociology from Ohio State University. For the past 30 years, he has been writing on and working in community-based projects in both the United States and several countries in Latin America. Most recently, he worked on a project in Ecuador that was devoted to building a health center in a poor community. Currently, he is a professor of sociology at the University of Miami. He is author of *Community-Based Interventions*.

Karie Jo Peralta is assistant professor of sociology at the University of Toledo, Toledo, Ohio. She received her Ph.D. from the University of Miami. Her present interests include community-based research and race and ethnic relations.

Jesús Ramírez is a doctoral student from the Philosophy Department at the University of South Florida, Tampa. He received his B.A. and M.A. in philosophy from San José State University. His academic interests include Latin American philosophy, critical race theory, and applied ethics.

Khary K. Rigg is an assistant professor in the Department of Mental Health Law and Policy at the University of South Florida, Tampa. He received his Ph.D. from the University of Miami and completed a postdoctoral fellowship in health services research at the University of Pennsylvania. His present interests include behavioral health issues and community-based interventions.

Kyle Rosenberger, MEd is a curriculum developer and course designer in Ohio University's Office of Instructional Innovation and Heritage College of Osteopathic Medicine. His current projects focus on the utilization of instructional design theories and technology for innovations in medical education.

Marco Shappeck is associate professor of teacher education at the University of North Texas at Dallas. He received his Ph.D. from the University of Illinois at Urbana-Champaign. His research interests include language contact, second language acquisition, language and aging, and linguistic anthropology.

Chantelle Shaw is a second year medical student at Ohio University's Heritage College of Osteopathic Medicine. She received her B.A. in psychology from Hampton University. Her research interests include social and behavioral determinants of health, community-based approaches to health promotion/disease prevention, and health policy.

Daniel Skinner, PhD is assistant professor of health policy in the Department of Social Medicine at Ohio University's Heritage College of Osteopathic Medicine. His present interests include the politics of health care policy, hospital-community relations, and health care for underserved populations.

Chapter 1
Introduction

Steven L. Arxer and John W. Murphy

The Relevance of Community-Based Health Care

In the field of health promotion, scholars and clinical workers are recognizing community approaches as important to changing risk behaviors and health outcomes for populations (Baker and Brown 1998). An emphasis on community-based programs in health care is, in large part, a result of a gradual shift from individual-level explanations of health behaviors to more holistic views of health promotion. Today, many recognize that environmental, social, and cultural factors shape individual and collective health. This "ecological" view presumes a broad set of influences and social-environmental interactions that shape health decisions and experiences in crucial ways.

Recent demographic and policy changes have also helped to increase the profile of community-based health promotion given the promise and potential of this strategy to address future health care needs. Clearly the United States has a rapidly growing aging population; by 2050 approximately 83 million Americans will be 65 or older (U.S. Census Bureau 2014). This demographic shift will have significant implications.

Frist, there will be a large number of individuals who will be entering government sponsored programs, such as Medicare, in need of quality and affordable health care. The cost of medical care is often higher for individuals age 65 and over (Centers for Disease Control and Prevention and the Merck Company Foundation

---

S.L. Arxer (✉)
Department of Sociology & Psychology, University of North Texas at Dallas, Dallas, TX, USA
e-mail: steven.arxer@untdallas.edu

J.W. Murphy
Department of Sociology, University of Miami, Coral Gables, FL, USA
e-mail: j.murphy@miami.edu

© Springer International Publishing AG 2018
S.L. Arxer, J.W. Murphy (eds.), *Dimensions of Community-Based Projects in Health Care*, International Perspectives on Social Policy, Administration, and Practice, DOI 10.1007/978-3-319-61557-8_1

2007), while the risk of falling, disability (Chen et al. 2009; Fried and Guralnik 1997), and dementia (e.g., Alzheimer's) increases with age (Alzheimer's Association 2010). Approximately half of all Americans who receive long-term care services are elderly, with the vast majority of national long-term care expenditures going to this population (U.S. Department of Health and Human Services 2003). Many have noted that supplying necessary management and treatment will be a major challenge for Medicare and other social services, in view of the growth in the number of older Americans.

At the same time, the population will consist of a higher percentage of racially and ethnically diverse people. By 2050, the percentage of the United States' population comprised by Hispanics will double from about 12% to 24% (U.S. Census Bureau 2008). The opposite trend is taking place for non-Hispanic whites, with a projected decrease in this segment of the population from 69% to approximately 50% (U.S. Census Bureau 2008). Of concern to public health practitioners is the increasing prevalence of chronic conditions, such as obesity and diabetes, occurring in all groups but particularly among minority groups. For example, the rates of these diseases are often higher and less controlled for Hispanics than for non-Hispanic whites and blacks (Centers for Disease Control and Prevention 2011). Another long-term care issue is cognitive impairment and depression, which Hispanics 65 and over are more likely to have than whites (Alzheimer's Association 2010). This trend is again particularly noteworthy given that the number of persons age 65 and over who are Hispanic is expected to increase (Vincent and Velkoff 2010).

Health care reform is also an important issue in discussions about access, cost, and quality of medical care. While the 2010 Patient Protection and Affordable Care Act (ACA) has opened access to health insurance to more individuals, many other aspects of the ACA remain in question. On the side of the government, the US Congress continues to revisit and debate the legality of the ACA, and repeated calls are made to repeal the program (Walsh 2016). Meanwhile, in the private sector, major insurance companies are beginning to exit the health exchanges established under the ACA, thereby raising doubts about the price competitiveness of insurance plans for consumers (Johnson 2016). The management and delivery of health care present significant challenges when considering that many minority groups, particularly Hispanics, are often the most inadequately insured group in the United States (Angel and Angel 2009).

The reality is that the needs of a diverse, elderly population will test the social service safety net of programs such as Medicare, Medicaid, and the insurance exchanges. Stanford (1994) noted some decades ago the impact of an older, more diverse population:

> as the older population increases and becomes more diverse, it becomes a driving force for changed required to meet the challenge of providing the quality of life we have come to expect. Aggregate skills and energy will need to be mobilized. Diversity as a social force will require us to consider how different needs ca be met .... Older Americans are no longer bound by locale as they once were. The diversity they have brought to many communities has caused community leaders to re-think the way they plan programs and services. They can no longer plan as if they aged were homogenous. Diversity as a social force will help

change the way bureaucracies perceive their roles and responsibilities and the way they operationalize their activities (p. 1)

While Stanford alerts readers to the pressing need to adopt a health promotion model that is responsive to diverse populations, traditional approaches to health care are increasingly understood as too limited in scope.

Long-term care presents state and federal agencies with serious problems considering the population changes and costs related to managing chronic illness. Traditional assisted living approaches, for example, have not addressed the needs of many minority groups who, because they are politically and economically disadvantaged, have reduced access to these facilities. Moreover, health organizations, providers, and physicians have not been able to slow the trends in obesity and other chronic illnesses.

Core to these issues are questions about the effectiveness of a traditional biomedical model. This approach places physicians and bureaucratic health organizations at the center of medical knowledge and care, but this strategy may be too disconnected from the growing and changing communities that they serve. In this context, community-based projects are thought to provide a more cost-effective and culturally sensitive way of delivering health care. In short, the resources and will power of the general population can be used to lower risk and prevent and manage illness.

This book examines the theoretical and practical dimensions of community-based projects in health care. Particular attention is given to how community-based programming can serve as a more appropriate model within the current demographic, social, and economic context. In many circles, a traditional biomedical model to health care has been critiqued. Additionally, community-centered approaches have been praised for offering a new perspective and set of solutions to emerging health challenges. But while community-based models are popular among public health scholars and practitioners who seek more participatory ways to promote health in communities, discussions often ignore what Alfred Schutz (1964) called the "deep assumptions" that underpin community projects. In the case of community-based health care, the philosophy that sustains notions of community, participation, and knowledge may be obscured without careful attention to the assumptions behind these ideas.

A central theme in the following chapters is that those who adopt a community-based approach can benefit from considering the symbolism that underpins their health care projects. The ways in which community, institutions, and knowledge are defined can shape the nature of health interventions. Public health workers, gerontologists, and epidemiologists are currently seeking a range of solutions to the problems confronting health care in the first half of the twenty-first century. However, the promise of a community-based approach to address these issues may go underutilized without careful theoretical examination. In particular, the subtle and historically relied upon symbolism of biomedicine may reintroduce elements into community projects that begin to limit the options and practices available to health promoters.

The Legacy of Biomedicine

The biomedical model emerges from the modern Western intellectual tradition. The cornerstone of this tradition is a commitment to a dualistic view of the world. Dualism is based on the separation of objectivity and subjectivity (Murphy 1989). With respect to biomedicine, dualism has taken the form of a commitment to a worldview composed of certain epistemological principles and practices. In this framework, health is seen as an object of knowledge. Objectification occurs in that health is externalized and understood to be a *thing* that can be dispassionately observed. In a Cartesian sense, knowledge is divorced from the knower. This separation, or dualism, is thought to be essential to the knowledge acquisition process, since this maneuver guarantees the objective status of information. Knowledge, in short, is based on empirical characteristics and not necessarily human action.

With respect to medicine, the Western tradition has focused on the use of positivistic and quantitative approaches (Katz 1996). The medical enterprise has been centered on observing and documenting the empirical conditions of the body. In this way, objective facts emerge to identify states of the body. A naturalistic model assumes that health (and illness) is material, located primarily in the individual where observations can be made effectively. Some argue that this model continues to be a "master narrative" in health care philosophy and action (Biggs and Powell 2001).

This portrayal has had various consequences on the conceptualization and delivery of health care. First, a biocentric viewpoint means that health care occurs at the individual as opposed to community level. Illness is something that is confined to the body (Powell 2006). The goal is to identify aberrations that disturb the normal functioning of the body and treat the individual in order to remove a problem.

Second, a biomedical model privileges medical experts as those who can accurately make health decisions (Blackburn 1983). A goal associated with epistemological dualism is for objective information to avoid contamination by interpretation or subjectivity. In this way, the mind can accurately perceive reality. Correctly observing the body means relying primarily on scientific and technical methods that minimize bias.

What is important here is that medical experts are imagined to be best suited to look for empirical signals, since they have been trained in the latest scientific methods. With the aid of technology that presents detailed information, the location of illness or disease is made clear. Good treatment decisions, therefore, are self-evident and unbiased. Conversely, nonexperts are marginalized in the knowledge production process. In this context, patients and those who surround them (family, friends, and community members) are viewed to confound the situation due to their emotions and interests. Without having the discipline provided by science, the idiosyncrasies of daily life would make health care unpredictable in the hands of community members.

And third, a biomedical approach has meant that clinical and medical settings have become the preferred location to offer health care as opposed to communities.

Hospitals, physician offices, and clinics are understood to be the most reasonable places to collect patient data, make diagnoses, and implement interventions. Unlike a patient's home or community, medical care settings are imagined to supply the necessary level of rationality to carry out science. Hospitals, for example, take on the nature of a bureaucracy. These places are run by formal, rigid guidelines and a hierarchy of positions. This formalization is presumed to provide a neutral space where experts can apply biomedical principles and practices in the absence of daily distractions. After all, hospitals are very different from the communities where patients live.

No doubt, this trend has been critiqued by a range of health scholars and practitioners. The turn to becoming community based is in fact a response to what some see as the problems endemic to a biomedical approach (Murphy 2014). For while medical settings are the focus of health care encounters, significant segments of the population are either uninsured or underinsured. Moreover, simply a biotechnical approach to health evaluation and treatment does not address the needs of an increasingly aging and diverse population. In both cases, chronic disease and the socialcultural factors that impact illness are beyond the scope of acute technical solutions.

As Karl Marx noted some time ago, alienation occurs when institutions are not responsive to human needs and persons no longer feel that they have control over their lives. However, a community-based approach is meant to restore the idea that persons can direct their lives through their own participation in key institutions. In the arena of health care, individuals can engage with those around them, deploy the range of skills found in their communities, and change their destinies.

Beyond Biomedicine: The Rise of a Community-Centered Model and Holistic Care

As a perspective, community-based health promotion is guided by the idea of primary prevention at the population level. Community-based programs, therefore, use various intervention strategies that target health-risk behaviors among individuals, groups, and organizations (Blackburn 1983). They also pursue policy and environmental changes designed to support positive health outcomes. These aims are accomplished by organizing health intervention programs that are integrative and comprehensive. Specifically, health care is not limited to medical care settings or the purview of physicians. Rather, community-based programs include community members and leaders, social networks, and communication and education strategies (Blackburn 1983). Community-based projects are said to emphasize holism by opposing a physician- and medical-centered approach.

The beginnings of community-based health programs can be marked in the 1960s with efforts to reduce rates of cardiovascular disease in the United States and other industrialized countries (Winkleby 1994). While early programs still used a biomedical model that focused on identifying and treating high-risk individuals, emerging research started to recognize the impact of behavioral factors (Kaplan 1985). A decade later, in the 1970s, heart disease prevention began to adopt a new approach that included programs focused on communities and encouraged the adoption of interventions aimed at changing environmental factors. Major-funded community-based prevention trials were implemented by the 1980s by the National Heart, Lung, and Blood Institute. The centerpiece of these programs was the idea that primary prevention and public health were more effective than clinically focused strategies at changing behavioral and environmental risk factors (Winkleby 1994). The Centers for Disease Control and Prevention (CDC) expanded the use of the community-based approach in the mid-1980s by emphasizing the development of volunteer community networks to assist in health promotion (Goodman et al. 1993). In the 1990s, the CDC implemented comprehensive community planning to prevent and manage HIV and AIDS (Holtgrave et al. 1995). And by the end of the twentieth century, the CDC's focus on individual "lifestyles" as a primary prevention strategy had waned in favor of a more comprehensive social-ecological model and the inclusion of communities as a way to modify social-environmental risk factors (Holtgrave et al. 1995).

Nowadays the idea that individuals cannot be isolated from their social context, and that successful health interventions must do more than identify and treat illness at the individual level, represents the core of epidemiological theory and public health policy. Community-based programs are, therefore, meant to overcome the position that health care takes place only in doctor's offices, hospital treatment rooms, and clinical laboratories. In particular, biomedical and clinical models tend to distance individuals from their own health promotion.

A key contribution of this book is a critical investigation of the popular ideas and strategies discussed above that are associated with community-based health projects. The purpose is to take community-based symbolism seriously and consider how further efforts should be taken to avoid the reductionism of biomedicine. Specifically, care should be taken to ensure that the dualism of biomedicine is not reintroduced into community-based discourse. Recent calls for more holistic healthcare practice suggest that both academics and practitioners should reaffirm the community-based perspective as a way to promote more culturally relevant and participatory health care.

Reaffirming Community-Based Imagery

Given recent interest in community-based projects, a reasonable question is what makes a project *community-based*? The literature presents a wide range of meanings and definitions of this term. Apparently, a project is community-based if specific ideas or practices are employed. For example, a community-based approach is said to be guided by community participation, empowerment, and agency. A standard typology of community-based projects often ranges from viewing community to be a setting or target for interventions to a resource and change agent (Rothman 1995). These concepts are certainly important for they help to frame the goals and intentions of a project; however, their appearance does not necessarily clarify the philosophical backdrop of a community-based approach. Participation may be used simply to increase involvement, while broader issues related to the structure of inclusion are ignored. Similarly, notions of empowerment and agency may be taken to mean that communities lack something essential that researchers and practitioners need to instill by providing knowledge and training to community members.

To better appreciate these ideas and their implications, their epistemological base requires exploration. While a more thorough review of these and other key dimensions to community-based approaches is forthcoming, the following aids as a backdrop to upcoming chapters. Some of the central philosophical assumptions of a community-based orientation include a rejection of the naturalism and structuralism traditionally associated with biomedicine and at times conveyed through ecological imagery.

From Social Ecology to the Symbolism of Community

To borrow from Lyotard (1984), a naturalistic viewpoint is based on "metanarratives." A metanarrative refers to an idea that is used to support key features of existence, such as identity, knowledge, or society. As the term suggests, metanarratives are grand accounts of how the world works. Their all-encompassing and objective character allows these tales to perform this vital function of sustaining reality. For example, in modern society, ideas that support a naturalistic and empirical view of the world have become dominant. Additionally, evolutionary principles of competition and a belief in science have helped to advance the notion that medical nomenclature and technology are ideal ways of organizing health care. An overarching naturalistic narrative has also been part of community-based health perspectives, namely, in the form of social ecology.

Consistent with the early work of Uriel Bronfenbrenner (1979) and other system theorists (McLeroy et al. 1988; Poland et al. 2000; Stokols 1992), an ecological orientation locates individuals within a broad social context that includes an individual's history, psychology, values, interpersonal relationships, community, policies, and cultural environment. The point is that individual behavior, and health in particular, is the result of many factors and influences. This perspective suggests that a wide range of considerations—such as social networks, families, and education—contribute to health outcomes.

An ecological viewpoint defines a community in structural terms. Similar to the social system of Talcott Parsons (1951), a community is understood to be a natural system comprised of parts (values, norms, and attitudes) that are connected through various linkages (family, social networks, public policy). As Stokols (1992) notes, a community environment represents "an array of independent attributes" and their "composite relationships" (p. 7). Although the intention is to acknowledge the complexity of a community, focusing on the structural side of this group may lead to problems. To the extent that a social-ecological model relies on naturalistic portrayals of community, this viewpoint may lead to new forms of reductionism that mirror those associated with biomedicine.

A social-ecological viewpoint presents what Wrong (1961) argued is an "oversocialized" view of human behavior. While presenting a more complex image, conceiving a community as ecological suggests that human efforts are directed by intractable structures. Parsons (1970), for example, argued that both natural and social systems have a hierarchical order that situates humans as being directed by societal directives. In this case, communities are transformed into an abstract system that misrepresents the agency of their members (Harris 2010). Thinking of community in a naturalistic and structural way, as a mélange of biosocial influences, is reductionistic and downplays agency. In short, the chapters of this book uniquely describe how a community is symbolic and constructed, as opposed to crudely empirical.

Community-Based Planning as a "People's Science"

Another relevant issue is the way that community-based planning approaches the knowledge production process. Although an ecological model presents the notion of holism, this approach does not necessarily place community members at the center of health projects. Viewing health issues, for instance, to be the result of a matrix of factors can certainly lead to a more inclusive approach that recognizes communities to be important settings, and even resources, in the planning process (McLeroy et al. 1988). Greater inclusion, however, still leaves room for communities to be marginalized when undertaking interventions.

Being community-based does not simply mean the adoption of a complex view of communities. Nor does this term mean that planners only need to work with or through communities. In this regard, communities are not empirical entities that can be catalogued and manipulated to achieve some end. In both cases, communities are treated abstractly, that is, as *things*. While an ecological model suggests that an empirical approach is the best way to conduct community-based research and planning, this form of knowledge production can be narrow.

Again, what is ignored is that communities are creative as opposed to empirical. Communities encompass the ways in which individuals come to interpret themselves and others (Puddifoot 1995). Therefore, a community-based approach does not reduce knowledge of communities to their empirical attributes—such as geography, race, unemployment rate, or income. To do so would circumscribe communities as predetermined and miss the interpretive nature of community life. As Pollner (1987) notes, communities are best envisioned as modalities of reasoning. This claim refers to the idea that a community represents the myriad of definitions and assumptions used by persons for dealing with everyday life. Community-based researchers, therefore, should take seriously these conceptual elements when making plans. In short, a social indicator, such as income level, does not determine health behavior but how this factor is interpreted.

What is important is that a community-based philosophy rejects the epistemological dualism found in science. Those who adopt an ecological approach, for example, may seek to increase the number of community variables in their studies. This strategy, in turn, leads to more precise measurements of community behavior and their causes. While the formalization and instrumentation tied to science may garner a sense of objectivity, community-based planners do not intend to achieve value neutrality (Fish 1989). As McNeely (1999) argues, central to the philosophy of community-based planning is that knowledge is based on community participation.

Because participation goes to the core of community-based planning, treating health as the result of a confluence of objective indicators presents a passive view of communities. The experiences of communities are not simply the result of environmental and social forces, but rather these persons interpret their worlds and chart a course based on this effort. In other words, communities define their needs and move forward with plans to solve problems. Most important, therefore, is that community-based projects foster this participation. Otherwise, projects are external to communities and do not embody the worldviews of their members. In this way, Fals Borda (1988) argues that community-based projects should represent "a people's science" (p. 93). What he means is that community-based approaches require a radical form of participation—namely, that the local knowledge of communities guides all health and any other projects.

Organization of the Book

This book explores central issues that can aid community-based scholars and practitioners in the development of their health-care projects. In this effort, the focus is on key dimensions of community-based projects. Some of these themes encompass more practical considerations, such as promoting community voice, the use of community health committees, the nature of physician training, and the adoption of community mapping. Other more theoretical considerations highlight the politics of knowledge production in community-based work, methodological considerations in data collection, and the idea that dialogue should be at the heart of medicine.

In Chap. 2, John W. Murphy examines the role of narrative medicine in public health. Historically, discussions about community-based health have been dominated by a biomedical model—an orientation that emphasizes the superiority of objectivity, scientific knowledge, and medical experts in health promotion. The assumption is that medical experts who possess objective facts have credibility and exclusive authority to speak about health in communities. Critics argue, however, that this form of epistemological realism fails to acknowledge the social context and local nature of well-being. Medical experts function in a vacuum while ignoring the community or social significance of health. The purpose of this chapter, accordingly, is to discuss the role that narrative medicine can play in elevating the voices and perspectives of community members.

Keeping with the theme of research in health care, Steven L. Arxer, Maria del Puy Ciriza, and Marco Shappeck consider the role of qualitative research in community-based health projects. Chapter 3 investigates the importance of using a methodology that involves community members in all dimensions of health projects and encourages them to become self-directed. An ideal approach has often been recognized to include qualitative and participatory action research. In both cases, the traditional renditions of knowledge, researcher, and subject are reimagined. Rather than a naturalistic approach, community-based research appreciates the cultural and social facets of reality. A naturalistic perspective sees reality as empirical and research as the collection of objective attributes possessed by persons or communities. On the other hand, a community-based approach rejects that humans are passive and reducible to empirical properties. Instead, persons should be viewed as agents who shape their identities and surroundings.

In Chap. 4, Berkeley Franz, Chantelle Shaw, and Keilah Ketron discuss the role health committees can play in democratizing community-based research strategies. Traditional methodologies are insufficient to generate holistic community-based projects. What is missing from both quantitative and even some qualitative approaches is community-sensitive data collection that helps inform social policies. In both cases, an asymmetrical relationship between expert researchers and community subjects is often maintained. At best, community members are "trained" as pseudo researchers, although this approach usually implies having these persons simply follow technical directives, such as deploying a questionnaire. This strategy fails to integrate community members fully into the research program and fundamentally direct the knowledge acquisition process. These committees not only include community members but encourage these individuals to direct, and even control, the planning process.

Chapter 5 is centered on the nature of dialogue between researchers and community residents. Jung Min Choi argues that dialogue should be the core of community-based interventions. Nonetheless, the history of these projects has had a realistic bias. Communities are thus divorced from the ways in which they define their social worlds and, instead, related to characteristics (e.g., race, gender, and other health indicators) that can be isolated and quantified. When conceived in this manner, communities are viewed to be things. However, this outlook ignores the social meanings that shape the self-definitions of a community and guide their behavior and decision-making. Community needs, therefore, are observed rather than understood. This chapter suggests that a community is not a composite of attributes but rather a modality of existence. Therefore, gaining entry into the linguistic or interpretive world of a community is necessary to produce relevant medicine.

Karie Jo Peralta, in Chap. 6, alerts readers to a central theme in community-based work—self-determination and empowerment. Community planners are said to operate under a new orientation that includes the cultural practices of residents. In short, communities want to advance their own agendas and have policies that are local in nature. Community-based planners face the challenge of generating plans in an organic way that is inspired and directed by community members and, additionally, that reflect a variety of knowledge bases and outlooks. This approach requires what Block refers to as "emergent coordination." Community projects, for example, are relevant only to the extent that they serve the goals that are articulated by local persons. In this way, the politics of special interests associated with select persons and perspectives controlling community interventions is overcome.

In Chap. 7, Karen A. Callaghan takes a deeper look at the well-known practice of community mapping. Presumably, one of the first steps in community-based strategies is gaining access to the world of community members. This task often includes discussions designed to identify community needs and steps to guide an intervention. In this way, communities are viewed as "targets," and precision is gained by locating gatekeepers and informants to direct practitioners in the field. This posture presumes a hierarchy of information, whereby some persons possess crucial knowledge and others do not. But community mapping facilitates planning only when plans emerge from local definitions of social and material assets. In this regard, true community mapping sees communities as capable of self-direction and knowledgeable about the services and resources they want and need. Community maps, accordingly, should reflect the stories that community members tell about their lives, aspirations, and resource utilization. This chapter emphasizes the need to include community members in supplying a picture of a neighborhood and identifying its crucial elements.

The training that most physicians receive focuses primarily on individual patients and their personal needs. The goal, accordingly, is to develop physicians who are "patient centered." In Chap. 8, David Laubli, Daniel Skinner, and Kyle Rosenberger consider how a community-based strategy is broader, is population centered, and deals with the social determinants of health. What this shift in orientation means is that physicians must be trained in how to work in communities, use a variety of intervention strategies, and appreciate the thrust of primary health care. These and related issues will be discussed in this chapter.

In Chap. 9, Khary K. Rigg, Douglas Engelman, and Jesús H. Ramírez look at how primary care involves the day-to-day medical services that individuals require. Primary health care includes the broadest scope of health care, reaching patients of all ages, socioeconomic backgrounds, geographic origins, and health issues. But when primary health care becomes community based, interventions move beyond a focus on increasing access to service sites and information. At the heart of community-based health care is a reconceptualization of health delivery and planning. Community-based health care does not simply expand access to health services but rather deploys communities to give direction to any health initiatives. Ignoring this realm of agency reduces health care to issues of delivery efficacy. On the other hand, a primary health-care approach is community based when health plans are designed from the ground up and reflect the everyday lives of community members.

In the final chapter, Steven L. Arxer and John W. Murphy reflect on the prospects of promoting more effective strategies to community-based planning. An embodied view of planning is emphasized that grounds community-based projects in the biographies of communities. Also considered is how a post-biomedical approach requires a critical investigation of issues of power, democratization, and change are important for the future of community-based work.

References

Alzheimer's Association. (2010). *2010 Alzheimer's disease facts and figures*. Washington, DC: Alzheimer's Association.
Angel, J. L., & Angel, R. J. (2009). *Hispanic families at risk: The new economy, work, and the welfare state*. New York: Springer.
Baker, E. A., & Brownson, C. A. (1998). Defining characteristics of community-based health promotion programs. *Journal of Public Health Management Practices, 4*(2), 1–9.
Biggs, S., & Powell, J. L. (2001). A Foucauldian analysis of old age and the power of social welfare. *Journal of Aging & Social Policy, 12*(2), 209–221.
Blackburn, H. (1983). Research and demonstration projects in community cardiovascular disease prevention. *Journal of Public Health Policy, 4*, 398–422.
Bronfenbrenner, U. (1979). *The ecology of human development*. Mass: Harvard University Press.
Centers for Disease Control and prevention. (2011). CDC Health Disparities and Inequalities. Report—United States, 2011. *Morbidity and Mortality Weekly Report*, 60(Supplement).
Centers for Disease Control and Prevention and the Merck Company Foundation. (2007). *The state of aging and health in America 2007*. Whitehouse Station: The Merck Company Foundation.
Chen, L. H., Warner, M., Fingerhut, L., & Makuc, D. (2009). Injury episodes and circumstances: National Health Interview Survey, 1997–2007. *Vital Health Statistics, 10*(241), 1–55.
Fals Borda, O. (1988). *Knowledge and people's power*. New York: New Horizons Press.
Fish, S. (1989). *Doing what comes naturally*. Durham: University Press.
Fried, L. P., & Guralnik, J. M. (1997). Disability in older adults: Evidence regarding significance, etiology, and risk. *Journal of the American Geriatrics Society, 45*(1), 92–100.
Goodman, R. M., Steckler, A., Hoover, S., & Schwartz, R. (1993). A critique of contemporary community health promotion approaches: Based on a qualitative review of six programs in main. *American Journal of Health Promotion, 7*(3), 208–220.
Harris, S. R. (2010). *What is constructionism?* Boulder: Lynne Rienner.
Holtgrave, D. R., Qualls, N. L., Curran, J. W., Valdiserri, R. O., Guinan, M. E., & Parra, W. C. (1995). An overview of the effectiveness and efficiency of HIV prevention programs. *Public Health Reports, 110*(2), 134–146.
Johnson, C. Y. (2016, August 16). Aetna will leave most Obamacare exchanges, projecting losses. *Washington Post*. Retrieved from https://www.washingtonpost.com/news/wonk/wp/2016/08/16/aetna-pulls-back-from-the-obamacare-exchanges/
Kaplan, R. (1985). Behavioral epidemiology, health promotion, and health services. *Medical Care, 23*(5), 564–583.
Katz, S. (1996). *Disciplining old age: The formation of gerontological knowledge*. Charlottesville: University Press of Virginia.
Lyotard, J.-F. (1984). *The postmodern condition*. Minneapolis: University of Minnesota Press.
McLeroy, K., Bibeau, D., Steckler, A., & Glanz, K. (1988). An ecological perspective on health promotion programs. *Health Education Quarterly, 15*(4), 351–377.
McNeely, J. (1999). Community building. *Journal of Community Psychology, 27*(6), 741–750.
Murphy, J. W. (1989). *Postmodern social analysis and criticism*. New York: Greenwood Press.
Murphy, J. W. (2014). *Community-based interventions: Philosophy and action*. New York: Springer.
Parsons, T. (1951). *The social system*. New York: Free Press.
Parsons, T. (1970). *The social system*. London: Routledge & Kegan Paul Ltd.

Poland, B., Green, L., & Rootman, I. (2000). *Settings for health promotion: Linking theory and practice*. Thousand Oaks: Sage Publications.
Pollner, M. (1987). *Mundane reason*. Cambridge: Cambridge University Press.
Powell, J. L. (2006). *Social theory and aging*. Oxford: Rowman & Littlefield Publishers.
Puddifooot, J. W. (1995). Dimensions of community identity. *Journal of Community & Applied Social Psychology, 5*(5), 357–370.
Rothman, J. (1995). *Strategies of community intervention*. Itasca: FE Peacock Publishers.
Schutz, A. (1964). *Collected papers* (Vol. II). The Hague: Nijhoff.
Stanford, E. P. (1994). Diversity as a social force in an aging society. *Diversity and Long-Term Care News, 1*(Pre-Summer), 2.
Stokols, D. (1992). Establishing and maintaining healthy environments: Toward a social ecology of health promotion. *American Psychology, 47*(1), 6–22.
U.S. Census Bureau. (2008). *National population projections*. Available at http://www.census.gov/population/www/projections/summarytables.html
U.S. Census Bureau. (2014). An aging nation: The older population in the United States. *Current Population Reports*. Retrieved from, https://www.census.gov/prod/2014pubs/p25-1140.pdf
Vincent, G. K., & Velkoff, V. A. (2010). *The next four decades: The older population in the United States: 2010 to 2050, Current population reports* (pp. 25–1138). Washington, DC: U.S. Census Bureau.
Walsh, D. (2016, January 6). House sends Obamacare repeal bill to White House. *CNN*. Retrieved from, http://www.cnn.com/2016/01/06/politics/house-obamacare-repeal-planned-parenthood/
Winkleby, M. A. (1994). The future of community-based cardiovascular disease intervention studies. *American Journal of Public Health, 84*(9), 1369–1372.
Wrong, D. H. (1961). The oversocialized conception of man in modern sociology. *American Sociological Review, 26*(2), 183–193.

Chapter 2
Narrative Medicine in the Context of Community-Based Practice

John W. Murphy

Introduction

Narrative medicine begins with a simple but important idea. That is, individuals and groups invent stories that give meaning and purpose to their lives (Charon 2006). These narratives, according to Charon, should be the focus of medical interventions, if these services are going to have any relevance. The basic theme is that these storylines are key to grasping how illness is understood, including the proper design of any remedies.

Clearly narrative medicine interferes with the traditional medical model. Whereas standard medicine is materialistic and is primarily focused on physiology, practitioners of narrative medicine claim that this emphasis is too narrow. Physiology, these critics argue, has a very limited scope and therefore obscures many of the factors that influence illness behavior (Foss 2002). In fact, without these wider stories, interventions are likely to be misguided.

In this regard, those who support narrative medicine strive to become holistic. A biopsychosocial strategy, as Engel (1977) describes, should be utilized. A similar orientation is adopted by those who champion community-based practice. Accordingly, advocates of both contend that persons must participate fully in every phase of an intervention, or the needs and aspirations of individual patients or communities will not be satisfied. In the absence of this connection, and the all-important local knowledge, illness will not be framed properly.

This desire for inclusion has widespread support nowadays. After all, many persons feel alienated from vital institutions, including medicine. Promoting the required participation, however, is not simply a matter of politics. In short, the proper philosophy must be adopted, so that the institution of medicine becomes

---

J.W. Murphy (✉)
Department of Sociology, University of Miami, Coral Gables, FL 33124, USA
e-mail: j.murphy@miami.edu

more participatory. Charon (2006) warns readers, in this sense, that narrative medicine provides a "new philosophy of medical knowledge." Community-based interventions, likewise, represented at the time of their inception during the 1960s a "bold new approach" to service delivery.

Additionally, since 1978 and the conference held in Alma-Alta in Kazakhstan, health care is supposed to be developed from the ground up, or from the community, in order to be effective in providing care to underserved populations (Hixon and Maskarinec 2008). In fact, many of the strategies that are now a regular part of public health care originated from this meeting. At the heart of this proposal is the expectation that local persons will participate directly in the planning, implementation, and evaluation of services. As a result of this change, relevant services will be identified, thereby improving program sustainability. On the other hand, communities will acquire the skills necessary to monitor their health and organize interventions. This announcement is certainly revolutionary.

The thrust of this chapter is to illustrate the philosophy, in addition to the practice, that ties narrative medicine to community-based interventions, particularly public health care. This task, however, is not merely an academic exercise. For the most part, narrative medicine has been implemented in hospital and other clinical settings, and this application should be expanded. And on the community side, narratives provide a nice metaphor for describing local participation. Taken together, persons may become more involved in their health care, thereby improving the delivery service to individuals and communities.

The Problem with Dualism

The standard medical model is based on Cartesianism, otherwise known as dualism. At the heart of this principle is the belief that knowledge acquisition can be divided into subjective and objective elements (Wilson 2000). Furthermore, the assumption is that with the proper training subjectivity can be overcome, so that objective facts can be encountered. Indeed, within this typology subjectivity is thought to cloud judgment and obscure reliable knowledge.

With dualism in place, for example, physiology can be viewed objectively and treated as a machine. Biomarkers, accordingly, can be adopted as objective referents that provide clear insight into the operation of this mechanism and the course of a disease (Hulka 1990). On the collective side, communities can be identified with social indicators (Land 1983). These so-called objective features, such as sociodemographic traits, can thus serve to pinpoint interventions.

Dualism, in sum, permits biological or social facts to be divorced categorically from interpretation. In actuality the point is to cast aside subjectivity, in order to secure factual information. Even when subjectivity is tolerated in traditional medicine – by recognizing a mind-body connection – this element is treated as a symptom of biological changes. And with respect to communities, opinions and similar subjective factors are never more than anecdotal evidence. In both bases, subjectivity is either dismissed or marginalized.

In narrative medicine and community-based work, dualism is challenged. Specifically, narrative medicine is an outgrowth of the "linguistic turn" in philosophy (Rorty 1979). According to this theoretical maneuver, the influence of language can never be overcome and thus mediates everything that is known. As Roland Barthes (1986) proclaims, there is nothing outside of language, such as objective health referents. Whatever is witnessed, accordingly, is enmeshed in a narrative that specifies the parameters of illness. What constitutes an illness and a proper intervention, in other words, are revealed only in these stories.

Community-based work, on the other hand, elevates local participation in importance. In this case, human action, or *praxis*, is believed to organize and provide social existence with meaning. Arthur Kleinman (1992), for example, contends that the result of this association is the creation of "local worlds." These regions are significant because they provide access to how persons define and will likely respond to illness. Becoming community based, in fact, requires that special attention be given to these themes.

A question that is foreign to traditional interventions is raised by narrative medicine and community-based work. Specifically, whose reality counts (Chambers 1997)? With regard to both positions, the focus is on the meaning created by individuals or communities. Illness cannot be conceptualized appropriately and thus treated effectively, unless the social and cultural reality of these persons is seriously probed. Therefore, some critics claim that these positions represent a move toward "biographical medicine" (Armstrong 1979).

Like all authors, individuals and communities create worlds. And anyone who plans an intervention must learn to read the biography written by these persons. In this sense, medicine has become an interpretive activity, with practitioners expected to acquire what Charon (2001) calls "narrative competence," that is, the ability to decipher correctly a local story. A disease is thus never simply discovered but emerges against a background of claims and perspectives.

In this sense, narrative medicine and community-based work are variants of "nonrepresentational philosophy" (Thrift 2008). Simply stated, in the absence of dualism, there is no autonomous reality to represent. All that is exists are contrasting interpretations that vie for dominance and recognition as normal and, with sufficient support, objective. No narrative merely represents but always offers an interpretation of facts. Even realists provide only a realistic portrayal of life. However, not attempting to represent a health condition, and the objective facts of a case, is a significant departure from the past.

A New Style of Practice

Unsupported by dualism, medical practice might change in many ways. Two are particularly noteworthy at this juncture. The first is related to an epistemological issue, while the second pertains to the organization of interventions. In terms of epistemology, following the rejection of dualism, local knowledge is the centerpiece of narrative medicine and community-based interventions. Values, beliefs, definitions, and commitments are thought to be crucial for understanding illness and the appropriateness of any cognate practices (Fals Borda 1988). Particularly significant is that serious input should be sought from individuals and communities in every phase of planning an intervention. In this way, the knowledge pool that informs personal and collective decisions about health becomes the centerpiece of this agenda.

In the early days, after the passage of the Community Mental Health Act in 1963, all treatment plans were expected to be multidisciplinary. In this way, a wide range of information could be sought, outside of the purview of medicine. Nowadays projects such as OpenNotes and OurNotes have been designed to allow patients to review their medical records and even make changes if necessary (Terry 2015). The basic principle is that accuracy is possible only when the perspectives of patients are incorporated into the medical record.

This sort of inclusiveness is also desired in community projects. At one time "cultural brokers" were encouraged to come forward and supply vital background information to practitioners (Lefley and Bestman 1991). Later on community advisory boards and local health committees were created to guide interventions (Newman et al. 2011). Again, the aim is to solicit in a systematic manner the local knowledge necessary to identity correctly a problem and effective remedies.

This epistemological maneuver, however, requires that interventions be reorganized. Specifically, individuals and communities must begin to control medical interventions, instead of the usual professionals. To paraphrase Arthur Frank (2010), regular persons, who were formerly on the periphery of interventions, are now the experts. Lay community health workers, such as *promotores de salud*, are an example of this trend. This involvement, however, extends beyond the usual consultations and partnerships. In this new framework, local persons should shape every aspect of a health project.

This organizational change makes sense given the importance accorded to local knowledge. Nonetheless, at least initially, medical professionals may find this shift disconcerting. Clearly they have the knowledge and professional status required to make medical decisions and have been traditionally allowed to control this process. Additionally, most lay persons have been socialized to accept the standard service hierarchy and make, at best, a few timid suggestions. The domination of the medical enterprise is thus difficult to overcome.

Even within this dismal condition, the changes suggested by narrative medicine and community-based work are not impossible to envision and implement. But medical practitioners must be willing to recognize that facts are not necessarily obtrusive, because these features are embedded in the stories told by individuals and communities (Bruner 1986). And the only way that these narratives will come to light is by including their authors in the overall design of interventions. Yet this involvement will not occur unless the conditions are established that foster their complete participation. Specifically, the knowledge local persons have about health must not be undermined by professional nomenclature and the medical culture.

World Entry

Individuals and communities create worlds through their narratives. Although objects are part of these domains, worlds are predicated on experiences. Indeed, due to the irrelevance of dualism, brute objects are unavailable. In the local worlds described by Kleinman (1992), only meanings are encountered, since nothing evades the influence of interpretation. A world, accordingly, is thoroughly coded and represents a meaningful arrangement of persons, events, and other personal and collective expressions.

These worlds, accordingly, reflect various, and often contrasting, perspectives or worldviews. Both individuals and communities are often the product of several narratives that reveal facts in their respective contexts. According to Erving Goffman (1974), these worlds prescribe "evidentiary boundaries." In other words, how facts are interpreted and evaluated may be different in each domain. Consequently, the resulting social conditions may prescribe very unique illness realities. Health habits, for example, reflect local customs that are enmeshed in the expectations of individuals and communities.

The discovery of facts, therefore, depends on successful world entry. Practitioners, clinical or research, must cross over into these regions, in order to gain relevant information. Hence facts are never obtrusive, despite any talk about objectivity, and must be coaxed into the open. That is, the world that is operative must be displayed and allowed to inform all data.

A world is thus never simply confronted. Likewise, no information is ever gathered. These metaphors do not capture world entrée, particularly the arduous nature of this process. This outcome can occur only through dialogue, which is not the same as collecting data (Gadamer 1996). A dialogical relationship, simply put, is much more intense than merely examining, even closely, an individual or community. Dialogue is a delicate relationship that requires finesse and sensitivity.

Dialogue is not simply a skill, reciprocity, or a strategy but a way of relating to individuals or communities. As described by Martin Buber (1978), dialogue is a mode of meeting. The point is not to become simply aware of a local situation but to grasp how this domain has been personally and collectively constructed. Practitioners must thus leave their familiar worlds and enter possibly very strange places. With narratives playing such a pivotal role in personal or collective life, dialogue could be referred to as a sympathetic reading of a local reality.

Dialogue and Reflection

There are some technical issues related to dialogue. For example, persons must listen to one another, seek clarity, and exhibit toleration. None of these practices, however, led to the epistemological entrée that is essential to dialogue. In other words, insight into how others are constructing their worlds does not necessarily follow from these activities. Something more profound is required than paying attention to patients or communities.

In the literature on dialogue, reflection is identified as a vital component in this process (Mezirow 1998). But there are different styles of reflection. At the lower end, persons merely ruminate about past events or practices. The result is that these elements are placed in a context and revealed in additional detail. At the higher end, and linked to dialogue, individuals become aware of how they frame events and behavior, along with the limits of these schemes. As a result of this maneuver, the transition to another world is possible.

Consistent with narrative medicine and community-based work, the mind is viewed to be active and capable of self-interrogation. Persons can thus recognize this mental activity, along with how the world is framed. As a result of such reflection, the boundaries of any frame are available for examination. Furthermore, because of this focus, other frames come into sight and can be viewed in their own terms. As Hans-Georg Gadamer (1996) says, frames are rendered vulnerable by this reflection – that is, recognized to be influential but limited – so that dialogue is possible.

With the parameters of frames revealed, the otherworld thesis is confirmed. That is, frames are exposed to carve up reality in various ways. Following this revelation, persons can appreciate the need to overcome their frames to understand the worlds of others. This type of meeting, according to Gadamer (1996), is a key feature of dialogue. In dialogue a horizon is exposed where one world ends and another begins, thereby enabling persons to be understood in their own terms. In this way, dialogue is truly a crossing.

As a consequence of dialogue, personal or collective narratives can be read in the manner intended by their authors. Along with this achievement, health care can be offered in the world, that is, within the realm of individual or community experience. Health care can thus be properly situated and integrated effectively into the lives of persons. But there are no hard and fast rules to initiate dialogue and secure world entry. What is required is that all expressions of health or illness be treated as intelligible and with dignity.

Medicine in the World

Following the rejection of dualism, narratives are everywhere. There is no escape from the influence of language, and thus interpretation, so that objectivity might be achieved. Even claims about objectivity are stories about value neutrality and empirical facts. The identity of individuals or communities thus represents an accumulation and particular arrangement of narratives.

Because everything is now semiotic, the desire for holism is changed. In the past, this term meant that increased data should be gathered, in order to present a broad outlook on an issue. Nonetheless, the problem is that these data were treated as objective referents, like facets of nature, divorced from interpretation.

In the context of narrative medicine and community-based work, this version is abandoned. A natural ecology, accordingly, is replaced by an ecology of symbols. What this shift means is that individuals and communities constitute a montage or mosaic of stories. These stories, in other words, hang together, are "loosely coupled," as Karl Weick (1976) says, but form a coherent biography. These stories "make sense" of the existence of an individual or community and thus should be read in their own terms.

Community-based holism, therefore, requires more than exposure to a wide range of data but a proper interpretation or reading of local biographies. In order to emphasize this transition, Kleinman (1980) contends that this interpretation should be guided by "explanatory models." Rather than natural, these schemes reflect how individuals or communities partition knowledge. These models are underpinned by the values, beliefs, and commitments of these parties and thus represent different experiential realities.

This move to include interpretation as a valuable considerations does not signal the abandonment of evidence. Nonetheless, this principle is clearly expanded. Hence etiology is not simply determined by identifying a cause and then tracing the various outcomes. Such a natural portrayal is anathema to narrative medicine and community-based practice. First, causes are not immune to interpretation, while second impact is not a natural consequence. Etiology is not this neat and divorced from local idiosyncrasies.

As mentioned earlier, dialogue and the accompanying world entry are required for proper interpretation to occur. The basis of an intervention, accordingly, should be the "illness domains" that are created by the narratives that are in place (Coreil 1990). The key implication of this phrase is that illness may be defined very differently, depending on the domain in question. For example, the nature of an illness, the path to treatment, and an acceptable intervention are specified by these realms and are not necessarily uniform and linked to a universal rationale. Evidence is thus localized.

Typically holism is the product of recognizing multiple risk factors and their interaction. Therefore, interventions are expected to be multidimensional. This usual portrayal, however, lacks an element that is crucial in narrative medicine and community-based projects. That is, these factors exist in narratives that tie together the worlds of individuals and communities (Gergen 2015). Narratives have an internal logic that provides sound information; data validity is thus a local determination. A proper intervention, accordingly, requires that such an undertaking be world centered.

Conclusion

In both narrative medicine and community work, the world is not optional, that is, a nice supplement to objective data. In fact, without dualism this dichotomy collapses. All that is left are experiences and the various ways in which these stories are prioritized. With no escape from this condition, how medical services are delivered must be rethought.

In the past, the claim would be that interventions should become patient centered (Berwick 2009). This shift represents a nice sentiment, since patients and their needs are the focus of attention. The shortcoming of this strategy is that these persons are often presumed to reside in a standard and uniform context. The impact of narratives, in other words, is not acknowledged.

A subtle but important change is announced by narrative medicine and community-based work. Specifically, interventions should be world centered! The introduction of the world, as discussed throughout this chapter, signals that emphasis should be directed to local knowledge and how illness behavior is interpreted. Rather than simply increased attention, emphasis should be placed on proper interpretations. Interventions, therefore, are not abstract but attuned to culture and other relevant aspects of local existence. Advocates of narrative medicine and community-based practice claim that this change should result in improved medical practice.

References

Armstrong, D. (1979). The emancipation of biographical medicine. *Social Science and Medicine, 13*, 1–8.
Barthes, R. (1986). *The rustle of language*. New York: Hill and Wang.
Berwick, D. M. (2009). What patient-centeredness should mean: Confessions of an extremist. *Health Affairs, 28*, w555–w565.
Bruner, J. (1986). *Actual minds, possible worlds*. Cambridge, MA: Harvard University Press.
Buber, M. (1978). *Between man and man*. New York: Macmillan.
Chambers, R. (1997). *Who's reality counts? Putting the first last*. London: IT Publications.
Charon, R. (2001). Narrative medicine: A model for empathy, reflection, profession, and trust. *JAMA, 286*, 1897–1902.
Charon, R. (2006). *Narrative medicine: Honoring the stories of illness*. New York: Oxford University Press.
Coreil, J. (1990). The evolution of anthropology in international health. In J. Coreil & J. D. Mull (Eds.), *Anthropology in primary health care* (pp. 3–27). Boulder: Westview Press.

Engel, G. (1977). The need for a new medical model: A challenge to biomedicine. *Science, 196*, 129–136.
Fals Borda, O. (1988). *Knowledge and people's power*. New York: New Horizons.
Foss, L. (2002). *The end of modern medicine*. Albany: SUNY Press.
Frank, A. (2010). *Letting stories breathe*. Chicago: University of Chicago Press.
Gadamer, H.-G. (1996). *The enigma of health*. Stanford: Stanford University Press.
Gergen, K. J. (2015). *An invitation to social construction*. Los Angeles: Sage.
Goffman, E. (1974). *Frame analysis*. New York: Harper and Row.
Hixon, A. L., & Maskarinec, G. G. (2008). The declarations of Alma Ata on its 30th anniversary: Relevance for family medicine today. *Family Medicine, 40*, 585–588.
Hulka, B. S. (1990). Overview of biological markers. In B. S. Hulka & T. C. Wilcosky (Eds.), *Biological markers in epidemiology* (pp. 3–15). New York: Oxford University Press.
Kleinman, A. (1980). *Patients and healers in the context of culture*. Berkeley: University of California Press.
Kleinman, A. (1992). Local worlds of suffering: An interpersonal focus of ethnographies of illness experience. *Qualitative Health Research, 2*, 127–134.
Land, K. C. (1983). Social indicators. *Annual Review of Sociology, 9*(1), 12.
Lefley, H. P., & Bestman, E. W. (1991). Public-academic linkages for culturally sensitive community mental health. *Community Mental Health Journal, 27*, 473–488.
Terry, Ken (2015). OurNotes Project to Explore Patient-Generated EHR Data. *Medscape* (Feb. 3): www.medscape.com/viewarticle/839154.
Mezirow, J. (1998). On critical reflection. *Adult Educational Quarterly, 48*, 185–198.
Newman, S. D., Andrews, J. O., Magwood, G. S., Jenkins, C., Cox, M. J., & Williamson, D. C. (2011). Community advisory boards in community-based participatory research: A synthesis of best processes. *Preventing Chronic Disease, 8*, A70.
Rorty, R. (1979). *Philosophy and the mirror of nature*. Princeton: Princeton University Press.
Thrift, N. (2008). *Non-representational theory: Space, politics, affect*. London: Routledge.
Weick, K. (1976). Educational organizations as loosely-coupled systems. *Administrative Science Quarterly, 21*(1), 1–19.
Wilson, H. J. (2000). The myth of objectivity: Is medicine moving toward a constructivist medical paradigm. *Family Medicine, 17*, 203–209.

Chapter 3
Qualitative and Participatory Action Research

Steven L. Arxer, Maria del Puy Ciriza, and Marco Shappeck

Introduction

Research has certainly played a significant role in community-based projects. In community and public health promotion, scientific studies are often regarded as a central source of information for policymakers (McGann and Weaver 2000). The results of many research projects are viewed as supplying basic information that helps scientists, community members, and public and private health agencies in their decision-making. In this sense, social research has been depicted in an instrumental fashion—that is, it represents a tool used to assist those most closely involved in community health projects. Even activists, who oppose the top-down nature of traditional health care delivery, give primary importance to the technical side of research (Friedman 1994). Statistics and data collection techniques are central ways that local realties are captured and communicated to the larger public.

While community health practitioners rely on scientific investigations to aid their projects, the foundations of traditional social research often remain hidden (Pollner 1991). What is often ignored are the epistemological commitments made by most

---

S.L. Arxer (✉)
Department of Sociology & Psychology, University of North Texas at Dallas,
Dallas, TX, USA
e-mail: steven.arxer@untdallas.edu

M. del Puy Ciriza
Department of Spanish and Hispanic Studies, Texas Christian University,
Fort Worth, TX, USA
e-mail: maria.ciriza@tcu.edu

M. Shappeck
Department of Teacher Education and Administration, University of North Texas at Dallas,
Dallas, TX, USA
e-mail: marco.shappeck@untdallas.edu

© Springer International Publishing AG 2018
S.L. Arxer, J.W. Murphy (eds.), *Dimensions of Community-Based Projects in Health Care*, International Perspectives on Social Policy, Administration, and Practice, DOI 10.1007/978-3-319-61557-8_3

social scientists but have implications for those seeking to engage in community-based health practice. This point should not be regarded as simply inconsequential philosophizing, for in the quest to arrive at community health, this issue has immense weight. In this case, traditional social research conveys an image of the social world that is incompatible with community-based projects (McTaggert 1991). Furthermore, for all their good intentions and efforts, those who want to provide an alternative to the present form of health delivery will be limited by the parameters of traditional research: for at the very core of mainstream social science research is a worldview that poses challenges to the aim of community-focused change.

Recent interest in a community-based approach to health promotion suggests that there are limitations to the typical way that health care is conceptualized and handled (MacKain et al. 2003). A community-based model is guided by a different ethos, one based on community participation, empowerment, and agency (Rothman 1995). At heart, the idea is that health is connected to the broad social, cultural, and material context where individuals find themselves. Given the social etiology of health, human action plays a vital role in a community's well-being (De Hoyos 1989). Community-based health planning, therefore, requires an inclusive disposition that recognizes community members as central to the planning process.

As will be discussed in this chapter, an important step in developing an inclusive health model includes how the research process is conceptualized and conducted. Put simply, community-based health research must be careful not to imagine communities in an overly positivistic fashion that sees these groups as empirical objects of study. Conventional quantitative and biomedical approaches that seek to reduce communities to empirical attributes, such as geographical location, are not sufficient to appreciate the way health perceptions and behaviors are constructed within a community (Charon 2006). While the formalization and instrumentation characteristic of biomedical science may offer precise measurements, community-based planners should consider ways to explore the qualitative meaning-making process individuals use to make sense of themselves and the behaviors of others. Community-based practitioners, accordingly, should solicit the deep participation of community members. What can be called a "people's science" should be a goal in community health projects (Fals Borda 1988).

Given this background, the topic of social research is considered important in community-based health projects. This claim is true not only because persons do research on community health but more important because the research process can foster an image of a community. In this case, what appears to be a purely academic activity is intimately involved in shaping social relations. For as will be shown later, positive science requires the formalization and naturalization of the social world that can lead to the marginalization of a community in the knowledge production process. Here "experts" who speak the language of science gain status above the voices of everyday citizens (Richard 1993). This chapter will explore traditional social research to expose its underlying assumptions and view of social life. An alternative method of social investigation is also presented that takes into consideration the qualitative nature of knowledge, which offers a way to democratize the social research process and align this activity with the goals of community-based health promoters.

Assumptions of Traditional Social Research

Traditional social research is the hallmark of the Western intellectual tradition. Specifically, Cartesian dualism is the defining characteristic of mainstream social science (Murphy 1989). Dualism refers to the philosophical maneuver that bifurcates subjectivity from objectivity and places them on two separate planes of existence while elevating the latter in importance. Given this backdrop, the primary focus of social scientists has been to identify objective information devoid of human influence. Overwhelmingly, truth has been disassociated from human experience, since this mundane realm is believed to be fraught with bias and inaccuracy.

Enamored by the Cartesian version of valid knowledge, social scientists view facts as the purveyors of truth. In modern-day parlance, facts are regarded as objective because they possess the distinctive imprint of reality. In the end, facts attain the status of reality as more concrete, empirical objects. Thus, as Durkheim (1982, p. 52) noted, social facts should be treated as *things*, which have an existence all together divorced from persons. This image of social facts parallels a theme that underlies the natural sciences, namely, that matter exists in itself. The assumption is that a totally objective world of matter, with a structure of its own, exists independent of the human element. Also, this assumption has fostered the idea that the social world represents a natural phenomenon, and, therefore, this facet of existence should be studied in a manner similar to any other empirical object. As a result, the role of researchers is to reveal the laws that regulate social life. This conclusion, however, leads social scientists to the same problem of the natural investigator: the discovery of regularities poses a challenge, since the human presence haunts the search for objectivity.

The difficulty in securing factual knowledge has led to an ingenious solution, one that has been regularly sought. In this case, the social sciences strive to develop an ahistorical knowledge acquisition process (Murphy 1986). This strategy means envisioning research to be "dispassionate," where the values, presuppositions, interests, and beliefs of both the investigator and subject are neutralized, thus preventing facts from being obscured.

This has been achieved primarily by formalizing the research process through standardization, hypothesis testing, statistical analysis, and quantification. Stated simply, using these techniques is thought to de-animate the research process because of their mechanical nature (Ellul 1964). After all, if social investigators have only to follow stepwise instructions and be technically competent enough to employ particular procedures, such as calculating a statistical correlation, interpretation appears to vanish (Homans 1967). At this point is where facts are thought to surface and "speak for themselves," since every effort has been made to prevent human foibles from infecting the data.

Dilemmas and Dangers of Traditional Social Research

Depersonalizing data collection, however, seriously undermines social research in that formalization can easily distort social reality. Distortion occurs because standardization advances particular reality-assumptions that regularly go unnoticed and unscrutinized due to their alleged facticity (Cunliffe and Easterby-Smith 2004). Indeed, these beliefs about the nature of social life can jeopardize a researcher's ability to understand a community. Specifically, because the social world is believed to be a natural phenomenon that should be analyzed within formalized rules, the situational significance of facts is obscured. The existential quality of social life becomes ancillary in a world that has a definite pattern of recurring events; in other words, the social world becomes a structured phenomenon that abides by the principle of cause and effect. In the literature of community public health a guiding principle is the identification of "high-risk" populations, with interventions decided on the basis of "risk ratios" (Kellehear and Sallnow 2012). According to this view, researchers should imagine communities to be part of a causal matrix represented by the direct and indirect effects of numerous variables.

The problem with this scenario is that a neutral and disembodied picture of existence is deployed that neglects the human texture of social life. For as phenomenologists note, the world is not a brute fact but represents a "meaning construct" (Husserl 1970, p. 113). Following Husserl's notion of "intentionality," the dualism that has distinguished reality from experience is undercut. Therefore, experience must be viewed simultaneously as reality, since human consciousness and any objects are always intertwined. Social reality should not be regarded as a lifeless *thing*, as dead objectivity, but considered a *lebenswelt*, or "lifeworld," since the world is born, or constituted, through human *praxis*. What is important to note is that the lifeworld is not a naturally disposed location but a symbolic dimension that persons create and simultaneously inhabit (Husserl 1970).

But while phenomenologists show that the world has meaning, and only meaning, traditional social scientists emphasize the objective nature of facts. This bias prevents researchers from grasping the existential fabric that comprises a community's existence. In this regard, normative social science strives to eliminate the impact of interpretation in the process of gathering data. Naturalizing the social world and prescribing the parameters of formalization have been the two attempts to accomplish this goal.

However, the social remains hidden, since a machinelike research process cannot appreciate diverse symbolism—that is, logic outside of that prescribed by science. In point of fact, those characteristics of social life that cannot be neatly quantified or standardized—such as the assumptions, values, beliefs, and interests of both the researcher and subject—are often neglected. Still, if the world is truly the realm of everyday experience where persons create reality through "meaning bestowing acts," then getting at the nuances of a community becomes essential for understanding that social body (Murphy 1986, p. 328). Yet in trying to be existentially neutral in their search for truth, traditional researchers talk about a hypothetical society rather than a truly lived association of people. For as Husserl (1970) states, the world is historical, in that it is "subject related." To ignore the human texture of reality can only lead to an abstract image of social life that is disassociated from experience. In such a world, facts may be treated as things and used to produce an abundance of precise information, but this knowledge has little relevance since it is unrelated to any experientially, humanly constituted reality.

A dualistic version of social research is not well suited to craft community-based projects. First, in depicting the social world as a natural phenomenon, normative research fosters the idea that natural laws exist. This assumption allows the principles and practices of biomedicine to gain uncompromising legitimacy. In this context, health is externalized since the focus of care becomes the strict observation of the empirical properties of the body. As Katz (1996) notes, this type of surveillance relies on quantitative techniques, since these are assumed to provide objective and precise measurements. At this stage, the practice of health care becomes fully *materialized*, in that the focus of research is the empirical features of both individuals and their communities.

A second point relates to the relationship between the individual and the organization of health care. Because traditional social scientists give primary importance to a structured image of social existence, themes of adjustment and assimilation are emphasized. Given a totally objective world, social reality is immutable and in the position to demand recognition. In the end, not to adjust to this reality is indicative of delusion and irresponsibility on the part of dissenters. The powerful language of the absolute has been at the heart of traditional health care (Weed 1998). In this case, physicians often speak of structural adjustments that individuals have to make in their lives to promote their well-being, such as changing their behavior or removing themselves from certain relationships. Such alterations are believed to be legitimate, because, as was mentioned, science represents the most objective, equitable, and efficient way to handle social affairs. And in view of the empirical nature of reality, medical experts and technicians are seen as best suited to control the direction of health care. With the use of novel technologies and information, medical practitioners are thought to be well positioned to make optimal decisions regarding diagnoses and treatments (Fischer 2000). Despite the imposition, persons may be inclined to adjust to these external demands because they are impressed by structure and objectivity.

Up to now, the point has been to show how traditional social research distorts social reality and in doing so supports a positivist approach to health care. The rest of this chapter is dedicated to reviewing some themes of an alternative image of social research. For example, instead of attempting to acquire pristine knowledge and create abstract schemes, the goal of this unconventional approach is to delve into the existential quality of reality and gain appreciation of this social construction (Charon 2006). This alternative approach may be understood as "social research undertaken from below," since this modus operandi signals the importance of mundane knowledge derived from the everyday experiences of people. This strategy has gained supporters lately.

An Alternative: Social Research Undertaken from Below

An alternative research approach requires certain epistemological commitments. The most important of these is adopting an anti-dualistic stance. Opposing convention, social research from below does not distinguish reliable knowledge from what is created by human experience. Because all phenomena are shaped by human action (i.e., meaning constituting acts), valid knowledge must also be recognized to emerge from experience. As Lyotard (1984, p. xxiv) suggests, social scientists need to express "incredulity toward metanarratives." What this means is that researchers should be skeptical of projects that seek truth divorced from situational exigencies. Considering the demise of dualism, the traditional distance that has been inserted between subject and object is no longer legitimate.

In acknowledging the pervasiveness of meaning, the social world fails to mirror a natural entity. For example, instead of being simply an empirical location (a house), this dwelling place is a lived "field of experience" (a home). In this example, social reality represents a linguistic habit: a situation that exists due to persons continually defining their worlds and interacting according to these socially born meanings (Lyotard 1984). This condition is the lifeworld of phenomenologists, a realm of human significance where existence takes place. And while the world may appear *as if* it is real and substantive in the Cartesian sense, everyday existence is the product of speech building on speech—that is, a linguistic invention (Barthes 1985).

Although knowledge is thoroughly mediated by meaning inscribed by human action, traditional social scientists make the mistake of trying to purge facts of their existential quality. According to Husserl (1970), this trend is unfortunate because experience offers the only access to a community. Before valid data can be generated, researchers must gain entrée to the lifeworld of a people, for only this realm contains a community's biography.

This change implies a research program undertaken from the standpoint of community participation. To be clear, the goal of participatory research is not to study the world via value-free methodological procedures but to merge researchers' interpretive frameworks with the image of reality generated by a community (Schutz and Luckman 1973). For as Viktor Frankl says, the thrust of any investigation is the "encounter," where an *I* (the researcher) meets to understand a *Thou* (the subject) (Frankl 1984). Social research should thus be viewed as essentially a hermeneutic endeavor, as opposed to simply a technical process, since the aim is to discover the *meaning* of data.

However, traditional social research equates technical expertise with methodological rigor. Because *technē* is assumed to be value-free and autonomous, researchers are thought to be put into contact with an unadulterated reality (Ellul 1964). Knowledge continues to be viewed as objective and simply waiting to be discovered. Capturing data in an unbiased manner, therefore, is considered to be the best way to gather valid information. In the end, acquiring technical competence is believed to lead to the truth. The mastery of technique is thought to produce the formalization and standardization necessary for this task. The idea is that by allowing technique to command all aspects of the research process, subjectivity is controlled and unable to disrupt the knowledge acquisition process. As was mentioned earlier, the goal of this sort of science is to transform methodology to a mechanical affair. Stepwise instructions are followed that supposedly require no interpretation. In this way, the image is created that a neutral medium is available to gather and handle data without contaminating this information base.

The problem, however, is that procedural refinement and improved technical sophistication do not necessarily lead to increased accuracy. For under the guise of value neutrality, certain assumptions are often advanced that are incompatible with the region investigated. These are the tacitly held beliefs about objectivity, for example, that sustain the culture of biomedical science research (Foss and Rothenberg 1987). But in the lifeworld, where persons actually exist, these concepts may be irrelevant. Moreover, if knowledge is filtered through unexamined assumptions, a distorted picture of a particular social situation may be produced. In short, the public's views and needs may be sacrificed in order to be objective. But what passes for objectivity may simply be an irrelevant picture of reality that is based on unverifiable values. Mills (1967, pp. 50–57) refers to this version of science as "abstracted empiricism." His designation seems appropriate, since the focus on technical rigor obscures social life happening on the ground.

Because of the situated character of knowledge, becoming value-free may be counterproductive. After all, what can be gained by adopting a so-called universal perspective when knowledge is local? In other words, a formalized methodological scheme may have scientific appeal, but this approach does not necessarily have widespread applicability. Indeed, formalized methods eventually run into problems that are brought on by the values operating in social life. Specifically, a person's lifeworld does not disappear just because of a researcher's desire to transcend values and become objective. Thus, because the lifeworld cannot be avoided, the methodology of social researchers should be value-relevant.

While formalization has been primarily emphasized, the new motif is "epistemological participation." Rather than trying to achieve objectivity, understanding the "basic qualifications of speech and of symbolic interaction" should be of utmost concern (Habermas 1970, p. 138). What is required is that the assumptions that guide persons' existence be revealed. Researchers should grasp the way a community interprets itself. After all, since facts are imbued with humanly inspired meanings, knowledge only makes sense in terms of the practical goals envisioned by persons. Thus, as Gadamer (1975) argues, the purpose of methodology is not to eliminate values but to encounter them in the right way. In this case, the right way consists of allowing the needs and views of a community to be shaped by the lifeworld, as opposed to traditional research protocol.

With epistemic participation as a basis, social research becomes epistemologically responsible. This means that since the world is not simply an empirical object waiting to be recapitulated by an expert, a method of description must be adopted that recognizes the constructed character of reality (Lyotard 1984). Thus, researchers must be concerned less with classifying the empirical traits of things and more with adequately interpreting phenomena. Adequate interpretation refers to when events are grasped in terms of how they are actually experienced by persons (Ingleby 1980). Experience, however, does not fall under the conventional empiricist definition, whereby sense impressions impinge on a passive mind. Experience in the lifeworld refers to how people attribute meaning to their behavior (Husserl 1970). Persons are not inert objects pushed into action by the pressures of environmental and physiological factors. Action precedes stimulation, since human intentions supply stimuli with meaning and, thus, significance. Therefore, simply surveying the world for facts is not sufficient to gain real insight. Truth must be sought in a community's self-perception that distinguishes reality from illusion. Validity is possible, accordingly, only when researchers illuminate the rules of meaning creation that sustain a particular community. This research is responsible and can emerge from below, because all the knowledge gathered embodies social praxis—that is, reflects how persons organize their lives.

Another key aspect to developing a more sensitive research process has to do with how relationships are understood. As was mentioned previously, social scientists have preferred to talk about structures when describing the integrated nature of the world. For this reason, researchers have sought to uncover the structural linkages, or causal relationships, that hold the world together (Parsons 1951). Often variable analysis is used to uncover these connections. The assumption is made that variables have an obvious link to the empirical world and thus are substantive in themselves.

This view engenders a reified version of social life, since the human mind is not understood to have any impact on how the social realm is organized. But again, a false dualism is implied, whereby researchers assume they can distance themselves from the process of variable analysis. Yet as Blalock (1984) points out, the human element is profoundly involved at the core of empirical research, since the issue of conceptualization cannot be overcome. Before any analysis takes place, the parameters of variables must be defined, which is fundamentally an interpretive practice. The point is that the nature of relationships must be redefined, or the role played by human action in creating the frameworks that gives integrity to the world will be obscured. As a result, causal or structural linkages may be better described as thematic relationships. Phenomena can still be related, but now they are "connected" at the nexus of overlapping assumptions (Schutz and Luckmann 1973). In other words, a relationship exists between various social factors when the rationale of one phenomenon is assumptively similar to that of another.

In sum, a research program enacted from below requires that the human face of a community not be masked (Lydon 2003). Since the world is an interpreted phenomenon, the implication is that social life consists of diverse perspectives. Thus, researchers should not attempt to cover up daily existence through standardization, since constructing a neutral mechanism is impossible. Moreover, using a formalized methodology to understand a community may lead to the lifeworld being eviscerated, as the nuances of a peoples' existence are not readily reduced to quantitative indices. Researchers, therefore, may seek to expose the acts that sustain the lifeworld. By living at the boundary or horizon of their interpretive frameworks, researchers may begin to recognize how the world is constructed by other persons or communities.

Conclusion

At the core of participatory research is an ethical imperative that is lost in typical investigations. Specifically, because data are not neutral or collected in a disinterested way but rather embody the social meanings of a community, the human integrity of facts must be preserved. Implied is that data should not be interpreted or used in a manner that violates their existential domain. This moral responsibility might not be fulfilled by traditional research, despite personal concerns for a subject's well-being (Murphy 2014). The reason is because value neutrality cannot respect the epistemic context of a community, since the values of science are substituted for the parameters of meaning that persons deploy to organize their lives.

This moral imperative should be acknowledged by those who practice health promotion. Supporters of participatory action research, for example, argue that the will of community members should be consulted and given primary importance when their well-being is in question (Cornell 2006). Yet this participatory principle is weakened unless community-based health promoters consider methodologies better attuned to the importance of human action. Traditional social researchers risk failure because of their penchant for the model of the natural sciences and view that this methodology is the best strategy for directing policies. In this sense, conventional researchers may not be democratically inclined, since they trust the rules of science and not necessarily the will of individuals or communities to guide social action.

This scenario can be avoided if health advocates do not become blinded by the allure of positive science, which can mask the role played by humans shaping the world. A community-based orientation should be capable of respecting a community's lifeworld. Once the foundation of an objective world is upset, the conventional structure of biomedicine loses some appeal. And as soon as the world is recognized to be replete with meaning that is contingent, there is no longer a place for epistemological and social hierarchies endemic to conventional social research.

Employing a new theoretical approach to social research should not be regarded as inconsequential. While pursuing practical dimensions of community-based research is important, rethinking the methodological enterprise is not anathema to this goal. Democratizing the acquisition, collection, and interpretation of data can play an important role in promoting inclusive community-based projects. In fact, community-based health care operates from this premise. From this point of view, social researchers look to the desires and voices of citizens to determine what is humanly possible and not the rules or logic of science. Otherwise, research may become socially disruptive, since data that are devoid of a human connection will be used to sustain social practices (Murphy 1986, p. 337).

References

Barthes, R. (1985). *The grain of the voice.* New York: Hill and Wang.
Blalock, H. M. (1984). *Basic dilemmas in the social sciences.* Beverly Hills: Sage Publications.
Charon, R. (2006). *Narrative medicine: Honoring the stories of illness.* New York: Oxford University Press.
Cornell, K. L. (2006). *Social epidemiology.* New York: Columbia University Press.
Cunliffe, A. L., & Easterby-Smith, M. (2004). From reflection to practical reflexivity: Experiential learning as lived experience. In M. Reynolds & R. Vince (Eds.), *Organizing reflection* (pp. 30–46). Burlington: Ashgate Publishing Company.
De Hoyos, G. (1989). Person-in-environment: A tri-level practice model. *Social Casework, 70*(3), 131–138.
Durkheim, E. (1982). *The rules of sociological method* (W. D. Halls, Trans.). New York: The Free Press.
Ellul, J. (1964). *The technological society.* New York: Random House.
Fals Borda, O. (1988). *Knowledge and people's power.* New York: New Horizons Press.
Fischer, F. (2000). *Citizens, experts, and the environments: The politics of local knowledge.* Durham: Duke University Press.
Foss, L., & Rothenberg, K. (1987). *The second medical revolution: From biomedicine to infomedicine.* Boston: Shambhala.
Frankl, V. E. (1984). *Man's search for meaning: An introduction to logotherapy.* New York: Simon & Schuster.
Friedman, G. (1994). *Primer of epidemiology.* New York: McGraw-Hill.
Gadamer, H. G. (1975). Truth and method (2nd ed., J. Weinsheimer & D. Marshall, Trans.). New York: The Continuum Publishing Company.
Habermas, J. (1970). Toward a theory of communicative competence. In H. P. Dreitzel (Ed.), *Recent sociology, No. 2.* New Cork: Macmillan.
Homans, G. C. (1967). *The nature of social science.* New York: Harcourt, Brace, and World.
Husserl, E. (1970). *The crisis of European sciences and transcendental phenomenology.* Evanston: Northwestern University Press.
Ingleby, D. (1980). Understanding mental illness. In D. Ingleby (Ed.), *Critical psychiatry: The politics of mental illness* (pp. 23–71). New York: Pantheon Books.
Katz, S. (1996). *Disciplining old age: The formation of gerontological knowledge.* Charlottesville: University Press of Virginia.
Kellehear, A., & Sallnow, L. (2012). Public health and palliative care: An historical overview. In L. Sallnow, K. Suresh, & A. Kallehear (Eds.), *International perspectives of public health and palliative care* (pp. 1–12). London: Routledge.
Lydon, M. (2003). Community mapping: The recovery (and discovery) of our common ground. *Geomatica, 57*(2), 144–145.
Lyotard, J.-F. (1984). *The postmodern condition: A report on knowledge.* Minneapolis: University of Minnesota Press.
MacKain, S., Elliot, H., Busby, H., & Popay, J. (2003). Everywhere and nowhere: Locating and understanding the "new" public health. *Health and Place, 9*(3), 219–229.
McGann, G. J., & Wearver, R. K. (2000). *Think tanks and civil societies: Catalysts for ideas and actions.* New Brunswick: Transaction Publishers.
McTaggert, R. (1991). Principles of participatory action research. *Adult Education Quarterly, 41*(3), 168–187.
Mills, C. W. (1967). *The sociological imagination.* London: Oxford University Press.
Murphy, J. W. (1986). Phenomenological social science: Research in the public interest. *The Social Science Journal, 23*, 327–343.
Murphy, J. W. (1989). *Postmodern social analysis and criticism.* New York: Greenwood Press.
Murphy, J. W. (2014). *Community-based interventions: Philosophy and action.* New York: Springer.

Parsons, T. (1951). *The social system*. New York: The Free Press.
Pollner, M. (1991). Left of ethnomethodology: The rise and decline of radical reflexivity. *American Sociological Review, 56*(3), 370–380.
Richard, N. (1993). Postmodernism and periphery. In T. Docherty (Ed.), *Postmodernism: A reader* (pp. 463–470). New York: Columbia University Press.
Rothman, J. (1995). *Strategies of community intervention*. Itasca: FE Peacock Publishers.
Schutz, A., & Luckmann, T. (1973). *The structure of the life-world*. Evanston: Northwestern University Press.
Weed, D. L. (1998). Beyond black box epidemiology. *American Journal of Public Health, 88*(1), 12–14.

Chapter 4
Health Committees as a Community-Based Strategy

Berkeley Franz, Chantelle Shaw, and Keilah Ketron

Introduction

Among the many truisms of community-based health care is that communities must be intimately involved in the conceptualization of problems, devising of solutions, and the execution and implementation of programs. While community members across the United States organize and collaborate on a number of levels, this activity is often ad hoc in response to specific and often fleeting concerns about pressing issues, such as environmental hazards, crime, or neighborhood blight. Deep investments in community-based health require something more along the line of permanent, enduring institutions. To be successful, such institutions must possess consistency, formal rules, continuous support, and participation, in addition to a shared mission.

For decades, such institutions have existed under the aegis of health or community advisory boards (CAB) and bodies with similar names but unified by a logic of community organization for health. However, despite their concern with improving community health outcomes, community participation has not often been the focus of these boards. In fact, only recently have critiques of existing health advisory boards (HAB) been formulated in light of important community-based principles (Franz et al. 2016). Other scholars have used the language of "health committees" instead of merely boards that are solicited for information but do not have much

---

B. Franz (✉)
Department of Social Medicine, Ohio University Heritage College of Osteopathic Medicine, Athens, OH, USA
e-mail: franzb@ohio.edu

C. Shaw • K. Ketron
Ohio University Heritage College of Osteopathic Medicine, Dublin, OH, USA
e-mail: cs709414@ohio.edu; kk285014@ohio.edu

power in planning or decision-making (Murphy et al. 2016).[1] Although health committees have become increasingly common in the context of community-based health interventions internationally, less is known about whether any health advisory boards in the United States are operated similarly to international health committees and are under community control. This study, accordingly, offers an overview of the current state of health advisory boards in the United States and provides a typology for evaluating community health groups according to important community-based principles.

One approach that is gaining popularity in community health projects is to form local organizations that play a role in planning and carrying out health interventions in collaboration with local government, academic, or health care stakeholders. Usually a formal board structure is established, and meetings are scheduled to evaluate local health problems, conduct or oversee any health research being undertaken in the community, and plan any new interventions (Newman et al. 2011). Health advisory boards can be facilitated by a diverse set of organizations including local community groups, neighborhood organizations, government agencies, universities, and hospitals, among others. However, this variation in the organization of health advisory boards makes it difficult to determine if such groups are comprised of local residents and require that their input be taken seriously.

Community-based philosophy is predicated on the principle of full participation and thereby suggests that these groups be under local control (Minkler and Wallerstein 2008). The result of this orientation is that local residents direct these boards, in addition to determining the missions of these committees. In some cases, the purpose of a health committee is to develop training curricula where research skills and other health knowledge can be transmitted to local residents, so that more persons can be active and comparatively autonomous in improving a community's health. For example, Sandra Crouse Quinn has argued that health advisory boards have a potentially powerful role to play in protecting communities who are often included in human subject research by radically altering existing views on informed consent (2004). Other research has emphasized train-the-trainer models as a sustainable method to ensure that health advisory boards can participate fully in research in their communities. In these models, the skills gained during training allow residents to train other residents, thereby ensuring that skills are developed in the community and become part of an enduring skillset, rather than limited to a group of professionals (Rosenthal et al. 2010). A variety of train-the-trainer approaches have been documented recently in the literature on community-based health interventions (Orfaly et al. 2005), including examples of health committees providing training on research methodology, skills for participating in interventions, and evaluating and communicating the efficacy of any programs developed (Wangalwa et al. 2012).

---

[1] In this chapter, we use the terms health advisory board, community advisory board, and health committee all to refer to community groups developed in response to local health concerns. Each of these terms is used in the literature, and therefore we use them synonymously in this chapter yet recognize potential theoretical distinctions between the names of these organizations.

Most of the literature on health advisory boards, however, has arisen out of interventions occurring in non-US settings. Initiatives staged in developing countries, in particular, provide a breadth of research on community engagement, including models and best practices for health advisory boards. A paper published by the Shoklo Malaria Research Unit on the Thai-Myanmar border, for example, evaluated past and present community advisory boards established as the Tak Province Community Ethics Advisory Board (Lwin et al. 2013). This board was established for the purpose of engaging the local communities to "obtain advice and establish a participatory framework within which studies and the provision of health care can take place" (Lwin et al. 2013, p. 229). At the end of their evaluation, several lessons are outlined for a successful community advisory board. They identified the need for flexibility, the freedom to change as a group over time, and the need for being realistic about the capabilities of the board in the present context. They also underscored the importance of adequately funding boards and argued that dedicated facilitators be cultivated and maintained (Lwin et al. 2013). Meeting regularly in order to aid the "group momentum and group dynamics" and coming together outside the context of the CAB in order to continue to build relationships were also determined to be important (Lwin et al. 2013).

Another study focused on the potential for community health advisory boards to advance research, particularly related to the efficacy of vaccines for HIV/AIDS in South Africa. The authors found that there was often tension surrounding the purpose of the advisory board and whether the focus should be on protecting the interests of the community or furthering the aims of researchers (Reddy et al. 2010). Other important findings were reported on the nature of community representation in advisory boards. Specifically in question was whether community leaders should be appointed to boards, local residents should elect representatives, or a combination should be used. The authors conclude that such challenges have particular implications for setting up health advisory boards that allow for authentic community participation (Reddy et al. 2010).

Among the list of recommendations that have emerged from a study in Lusaka, Zambia, are training board members and identifying these persons in the community, both of which were related to the success of a committee (Mwinga and Moodley 2015). Training focused on understanding disease concepts, while medical research was found to be imperative for effective community engagement (Cheah et al. 2010). Possible hindrances to CAB effectiveness in the global health committee literature are low commitment levels and limited resources (Mwinga and Moodley 2015).

A scholarly literature has begun to develop on the utility of health advisory boards for community-based projects in the United States. In some cases, these bodies have explicitly made community control of research within their neighborhoods and involving community members a focus. Newman and colleagues (2011), for example, define community advisory boards as groups that are representative of the community in question and share "interest, identity, illness experience, history, language or culture" (Newman et al. 2011, p. 1). These authors distinguish clearly between traditional health advisory boards and their community-based counterparts and provide a list of best practices for forming these groups, including identifying a shared purpose, recruiting local residents, setting an appropriate governance structure, ensuring community control, and facilitating their regular evaluation.

Other studies on health advisory boards in the United States have focused on the challenges to developing community-based committees. When evaluating successful relationships and partnerships to advance community health, studies have identified several challenges that can be encountered. For example, professionals that collaborate on health advisory boards may not be used to or willing to give up control to local residents, community members may not have experience speaking about local health concerns, and neither group may have the skills to co-facilitate boards with a formal structure and rules (Holden et al. 2016, p. 5). Another study emphasized challenges in co-determining and communicating the shared mission of an advisory board and in effectively utilizing the strengths of community members who sit on an advisory board (Walsh et al. 2015).

Another case study on health advisory boards in the United States documented the process of transitioning from a traditional HAB to a community-based committee. In Harlem, New York, an urban research center was developed in order to establish a partnership between community members and local researchers. A Center for Urban Epidemiologic Studies was established in order to conduct research on the health of the city residents and promote "research collaborations" among institutions in New York City (Galea et al. 2001). Important lessons from this experience included the priority of developing a dialogue and engaging a dedicated core group in order to build a meaningful relationship between researchers and community members (Galea et al. 2001, p. 537). Despite early turnover at the community advisory board (CAB) meetings, eventually an ongoing dialogue became the glue that allowed the board to retain membership and remain viable (Galea et al. 2001, p. 537). Especially important was the "growing appreciation of the advantages of collaborative work and the role that collaborative work played in addressing social factors that affect health" (Galea et al. 2001). The authors of this study also emphasized the importance of continued education of both researchers and residents in CABs. This finding highlights a willingness of both parties to glean new insight for the betterment of the community. These authors identify the need for researchers to learn about a community's culture, as well as community members becoming familiar with the methods of research such as "protocols, institutional review board procedures and the conventions of empirical research" (Galea et al. 2001).

Although the literature on health advisory boards has been connected to community participation and the affinity with community-based participatory research (CBPR), little theoretical work has been done on the key principles of community-based philosophy and how health advisory boards would have to be structured to facilitate full participation of community members. Accordingly, below are four important facets of community-based philosophy, in order to provide a framework for evaluating health advisory boards that are currently operating in the United States.

Becoming Community Based: Local Knowledge, Dialogue, Full Participation, and Autonomy

Community-based philosophy is predicated on the idea that knowledge is fully interpretive. This principle suggests that meanings arise out of particular communities and can only be understood by gaining entrée to a particular setting. In the context of health, for example, symptoms, diagnoses, and interventions are not universally defined but instead take on a variety of local meanings. The causes of high blood pressure, for example, are defined differently in various contexts, and therefore sociological factors such as discrimination, and not simply psychological factors, are important for designing preventive practices and interventions that local persons find relevant and practical (Blumhagen 1980; Williams and Neighbors 2001). The sociological and anthropological study of illness has further pointed out that pain is both experienced and displayed differently depending on a variety of factors (Zola 1966; Encandela 1993).

Any interventions aimed at addressing local health concerns must be sensitive to the perspectives that are operative in a community if they are to be successful. This approach emphasizes the importance of engaging fully a community when attempting to design health care services and interventions that local residents will accept and find meaningful. The acknowledgment that health and illness are socially defined, therefore, requires community members to be intimately involved with improving health because information about the meaning that health has in a particular context can be shared only through this involvement.

This process of entering the life-world of local persons is often referred to as "dialogue" (Friedman 1992). The thrust of this second principle is to open a process of communication whereby interlocutors attempt to clarify one another's intentions and understand different perspectives. In community health, dialogue requires accepting that residents and the communities they inhabit may have values and opinions that are relevant to promoting wellness. Instead of doctors, city planners, or health departments directing community health interventions in accordance with standardized models, community members should direct this process. After all, if the goal of improving medical care is to assist populations and intervene before the onset of illness, information about the quality of life within a community will need to be expressed by local residents. When planners and other professionals attempt to understand local perspectives, solutions that are compatible with the daily lives of community members become possible.

In addition to learning to understand the meanings and definitions that are accomplished within communities, community health planners must also recognize the utility of partnering with local residents. The third principle of full and authentic participation suggests that community members must be involved with planning, implementing, and maintaining programs (Cornwall and Jewkes 1995). The goal is to fully integrate local knowledge into interventions that aim to improve population health. A key challenge in accomplishing full participation is that planners and other professionals have to get to know local communities and trust that laypersons can help direct changes in health, including assessing current needs, planning interventions, and evaluating changes.

A key implication is that community health professionals no longer possess the only or even most relevant information. For example, community members are more likely to find solutions that are considered to be practical, ensure that residents adhere to preventive practices, and identify with interventions (Shediac-Rizkallah and Bone 1998). Community-based programs are thus thought to be truly sustainable because residents decide the scope and structure of projects, participate in their implementation, and evaluate their results.

Finally, the future of community health must involve a return of control to local communities. This final principle – autonomy – underscores the importance of transferring the ownership of health care away from public officials, planners, and professional practitioners to community members. Such an emphasis recalls that the traditional mission of health care is to improve the lives of persons. When viewed from this perspective, health care belongs to the communities whose lives and well-being are at stake. Although many patients have been empowered recently through concepts such as patient-centered care (Pelzang 2010), true community autonomy in planning health interventions does not always follow. Authentic autonomy involves a deliberate shift to allow local knowledge and perspectives to guide improvements in local health. This change poses a challenge to traditional professional and medical authority and is therefore controversial. But improving community health relies on the ability of local planners to recognize the knowledge and skills held by communities and relinquish the power and control inherent to standard community planning.

The principle of autonomy is particularly significant, since authentic ownership allows communities to develop and pass on the skills required to organize and carry out medical care initiatives (Butterfoss 2007). When professional planners control most aspects of interventions, even when substantial neighborhood input is sought, local residents are dependent on institutions and are not able to control fully a course of action. Further, when projects or programs end and experts leave, local communities are often left without the training and power to organize, communicate, and address future problems. In other words, although short-term results might be improved by planners merely working in communities, community health improvement becomes sustainable when interventions are truly community based. These four principles can be used to evaluate the extent to which existing health advisory boards are community based and, therefore, potentially important for creating sustainable changes in health. Based on these principles, three guiding research questions emerged in the present study to help understand the current state of health advisory boards in the United States.

Research Questions and Methods

1. How are health committees and advisory boards organized in the United States?
2. Are these bodies truly community based?
3. What role do these planning groups play in community health interventions and evaluation?

In order to understand the current landscape of health advisory boards in the United States, a systematic web search of existing groups was conducted. To identify boards, a variety of keyword combinations were utilized related to health and well-being, the organizing body, and the structure of the group. Keywords related to health and well-being included health, wellness, well-being, preventative/preventive, medicine, and medical. Keywords related to the organizing body or location of the group included community, neighborhood, and local. Keywords related to the structure of the group included committee, board, task force, working group, steering, committee, commission, council, and advisory board. Four researchers participated in a web search using these search terms that identified 47 existing boards.

After identifying each board, a dataset was developed to document specific features of each board. The criteria used to assess each group included the meeting location, method of agenda setting, governance structure, history of committees, membership criteria, current projects, resident involvement in research, how and if minutes are recorded, participation in evaluation, partnerships with community organizations, official affiliation with institution, frequency of meetings, years in service, mission statement, whether and how minutes are publicly disseminated, and method of advertising meetings.

Information was collected initially from examining the websites for each group. Contact information was recorded for each board, and phone calls and emails were conducted to retrieve information that was not available on websites. Some contact persons were not amenable to such requests or were not able to be reached; this information is presented as "unknown" in the findings.

Findings

This web-based study yielded results for 47 HABs nationally. The distribution of these HABs included committees in 22 states and Washington, DC. Although each health advisory board was assessed on a large number of criteria, the focus here is on key differences with respect to community-based philosophy: committee membership, governance structure, frequency of meetings, formal affiliation, and current projects.

Committee Membership

Among the 47 health committees that were examined, three different qualifications were found to determine membership: residency in a certain neighborhood or region, appointment to committee board, and membership open to the general public. Of the 47 boards, 33% (15) based membership on residency status, while another 39% (18) used an appointment process to establish membership. Only 9% (4) of the boards had membership that was explicitly open to all interested persons. Twenty-two percent (10) of boards did not have this information publicly available.

Membership criteria

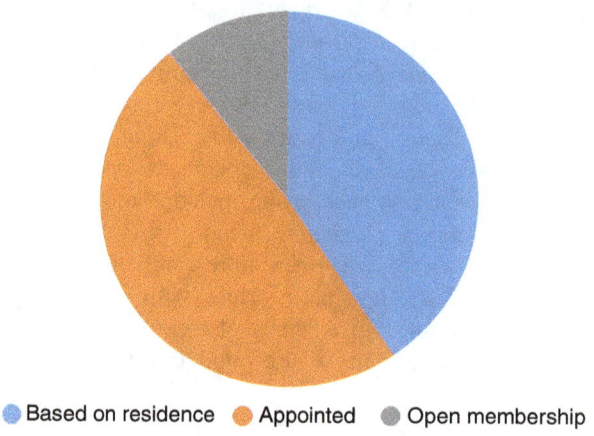

Governance Structure

There was comparatively less information available on the governance structure of health advisory boards, with 35% (16) not displaying details related to governance structure on webpages. Among those that did provide bylaws or specific information regarding the structure of governance, the majority were split between having co-chairs or a chair and vice-chair, multi-member governance (more than two individuals), and a flexible membership structure. Forty-eight percent (22) had two representative leaders, 15% (7) had more than three representative leaders, and 2% (1) had a flexible membership structure.

Governance structure

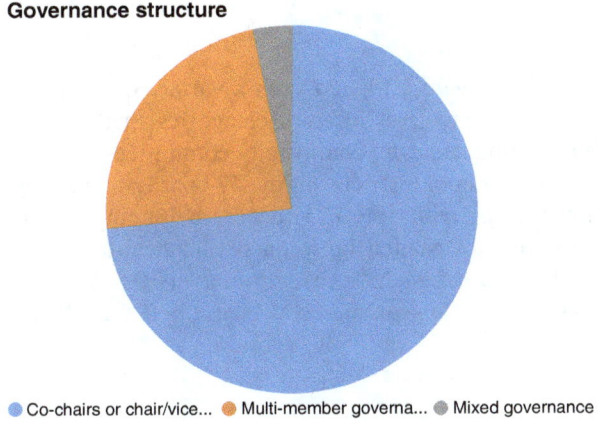

● Co-chairs or chair/vice... ● Multi-member governa... ● Mixed governance

Meeting Frequency

Information was most readily available regarding the meeting schedule of groups with only 13% of boards missing this information. Although meeting schedules varied significantly, they can be classified into four broad categories: monthly, quarterly, none of the above but <6 times a year (e.g., twice a year), or none of the above but >6 times a year (e.g., biweekly or every other month). Of the 47 boards, 30% (14) meet monthly, 35% (16) meet quarterly, 4% (2) meet less than six times a year but not monthly or quarterly, and 20% (9) meet greater than six times a year, but not monthly or quarterly.

Frequency of meetings

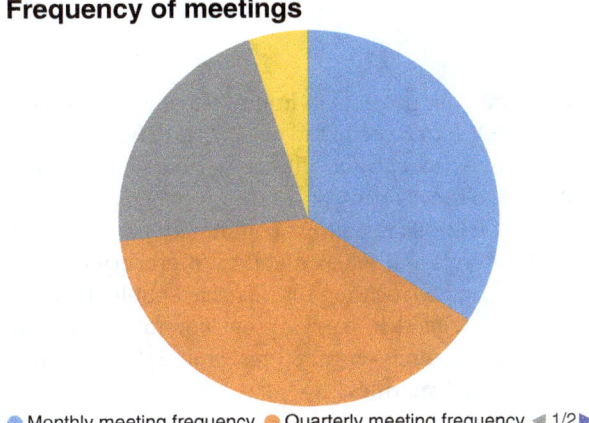

● Monthly meeting frequency ● Quarterly meeting frequency ◄ 1/2 ►

Affiliation

The health advisory boards identified were affiliated with a variety of different organizing bodies. These bodies fall into five different categories that include affiliations with public health departments, state, county, city committees, universities, community organizations, and school districts. Of the 47 boards, a majority are run out of city/state/county offices, with 53% (25) boards belonging to this category. The remaining boards are distributed between public health departments, with 17% (9) associated with boards, 13% (6) with universities, 13% (6) with community organizations, and 1, or approximately 1 board, or 2% affiliated with a school district.

Organizing body

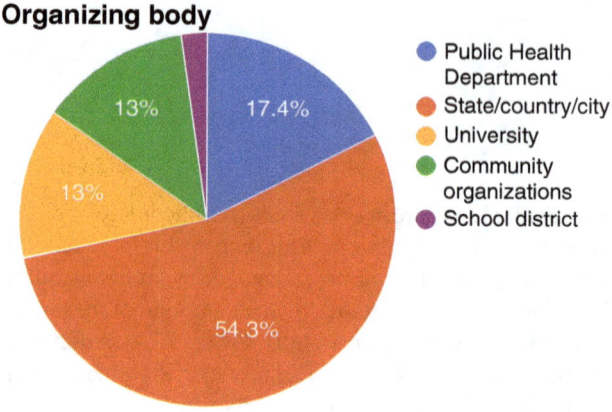

Diversity of Projects

Many of the boards have been involved with projects to improve the health of their communities. Most of these projects fell into three broad categories. The first category was health promotion, which included chronic illness and other preventive health education, tobacco cessation, and other forms of behavior change programs. The second category consisted of interventions to address community needs, which included improving access to healthy foods and the availability of grocery outlets, participating in urban design planning, and advocating for increased public funding for health projects. The final category related to carrying out community health research such as needs assessments, community-engaged research collaborations, and investigations to address local health disparities.

Discussion

From these findings several structural elements of HABs can be distinguished that have important implications for community-based health. In particular, the key point is that a typology of health advisory board features can be created that will allow health advisory boards to be evaluated with regard to the extent that they promote the participation of local residents, as well enact other community-based principles.

Governance Structure

First, several points can be made regarding governance structure. For example, of particular interest in this study is how different boards run their meetings. The most popular approach was to have two chairs, or a chair and vice-chair, usually drawn from lay community members, appointed to either two, three, four, or indefinite terms.[2] Although a significant number of boards appear to have been established by local public health departments, many report being established endogenously, often by community members themselves who met to discuss issues and ended up formalizing their board status.

Although there is not a single type of governance structure that is compatible with a community-based health advisory board, several considerations are important. For example, co-chairs could be a mix of community members and professionals to ensure buy-in from various stakeholders. Co-ownership may be important for the success of health advisory boards, if this organizational strategy facilitates mutual education between professionals or academic researchers and local residents (Quinn 2004). Establishing this relationship as a structural feature of all HABs intended to promote an equality of representation would constitute a palpable step toward ensuring that HABs are truly representative of and sensitive to community perspectives. Furthermore, rotating chairs would also ensure that conversations, agendas, and even the broader ethos of the board remain fresh. Ensuring that appointments are short- or medium-term, instead of the long-term appointments adopted by many boards, might also promote participation.

Agenda Setting/Minute Recording/Advertising

Although comprehensive data on agenda setting within HABs was not found, agendas appear most often to be established by protocols under Roberts Rules of Order, with agenda items proposed by chairs in advance, with an opportunity for additions

---

[2] Based on our experience with HABs in Columbus, Ohio, the preference for indefinite chair appointments is likely a function of the difficulty in recruiting and maintaining HAB leadership.

by HAB members. For HABs to fully allow for community participation and control, agendas should include significant input from local residents. While residents may serve as chairs who set the agenda, allowing input from both members and nonmembers will increase the diversity of perspectives integrated into discussions and allow control to remain with local residents, rather than only community leaders or the most active community members.

Similarly, many HABs appear to maintain minutes of each board meeting, but the internet search indicated that minutes are rarely made available on HAB web sites and even less rarely presented in a comprehensive manner. Additionally, information was largely unavailable that specifies which member of the HAB takes minutes or the procedures for approving and correcting these documents. This information may have a lot to do with who participates. For example, if minutes are taken by a community planner or other professional, notetaking may be relegated to including official agenda items or reflecting the perspectives of elites. Furthermore, making sure that minutes are available to local residents, regardless of whether they are members of the HAB, is important so that members of the community can understand the thrust of interventions being planned and provide alternative perspectives if necessary.

Finally, the extent to which HAB meetings are advertised to local residents is unclear for most American HABs. What information does exist suggests that advertising is often undertaken either by word of mouth, email lists, or fliers posted at community centers, health departments, or other central locations. Although more information is needed regarding how current HABs are communicating meeting schedules, advertising has important implications for community participation. If advertising is not undertaken carefully, many local residents may not know about upcoming meetings or may not know that their presence is welcomed. Furthermore, the type of communication used may mean that certain residents are more likely to know about board meetings and therefore get involved. To ensure that residents with different technological resources and skills, occupations, and residential locations within a community are included, advertising should be undertaken in a variety of formats. For example, meetings could be communicated by mailing and posting of flyers, emails, postings on online community discussion boards, and by word of mouth.

Membership

There are a number of ways membership guidelines can be established. The most common, of course, is based on location of residence, especially within certain zip codes or other neighborhood boundaries that may or may not conform to official definitions of the community. Other conceptualizations may focus on people who are invested in a neighborhood, who work but do not live there, or other committed citizens for reasons not captured by this category. In some cases, as with the Contra Costa Public and Environmental Health Advisory Board, which contains members from various neighborhoods to address environmental health concerns, or the Chinese Healthy Aging Community Advisory Board, which is invested in improving well-being among Chicago's Chinese communities, membership is based on a shared focus instead of residential status. In boards that transcend a single neighborhood or community, membership might cohere around communities of similarly situated individuals, such as those within a city concerned about environmental hazards (lead in water, housing stock struggling with asbestos removal, occupational hazards that united certain industrial sectors, and environmental issues based on shared geographies such as air quality or waterways, to name just a few of many possibilities).

Regardless of whether membership is based on geographical status or transcends multiple areas, the principle of open membership is important to ensure full community participation. These findings suggest that many health advisory boards currently operating rely on an application or appointment process rather than allowing all residents or concerned individuals to join. Most important is that lay community members are able to participate fully and play a strong role in all of the board activities. Due to the time investment of such participation, one option may be to provide stipends for this involvement. One challenge of maintaining community participation mentioned in the literature relates to achieving resident buy-in and willingness to continue attending meetings over time. Providing stipends to residents may help address this challenge, along with maintaining an open membership structure.

Frequency of Meetings

The frequency of meetings ranged from every other week to twice a year. The majority of meetings occurred either monthly or quarterly and no meetings occurred weekly. Meeting frequency, however, has important implications for the type of work that can be carried out by a HAB and the quality of local participation. If residents are volunteering time to participate on a committee, frequent meetings may be difficult to maintain without compensation. Incentives will be important for health advisory boards that wish to take on significant interventions or research. Ultimately, the purpose of the board will determine how often meetings should occur. But if health advisory boards are envisioned to be active and effective bodies capable of assessing problems, planning interventions, and evaluating and communicating changes to a community, frequent meetings and compensation for residents should be an important consideration.

Affiliation

If the goal of a health advisory board is to produce research and interventions that result in policy changes, community organizations may not be able to accomplish this aim without challenging the power of local governmental or academic institutions. However, boards that are not formally affiliated with any institution may have more control over the mission of the group and input into other features such as governance structure and membership. Moreover, if HABs are affiliated with just one institution, the focus of the board may be directly related to the mission of that particular institution, such as a public health department, and may be less flexible in taking into account local perspectives on health and illness. Finally, the affiliation of health advisory boards may have implications for how power is distributed among professionals and local residents. The bylaws may provide insight into whether the board is able to maintain independence from the institution, allow members to control resources, and direct the focus of any research and interventions.

Projects

The types of projects undertaken by HABs vary considerably from carrying out community health needs assessments to advocating for policy changes such as requiring nutrition information on menus or improved crime surveillance in a community. From the perspective of community-based philosophy, the types of projects may be less consequential than whether health advisory boards facilitate the participation of local residents and are active in addressing locally defined concerns in a community. Of particular interest in assessing current boards is whether a record of such activity is evident, and community members are able to summon the resources necessary to develop and carry out needed interventions.

What's in a Name?

The findings of this study suggest that although many committees share similar names, there is considerable diversity with regard to community participation in and control of these boards. For example, the most common names include some variation of "health advisory board" or "community advisory board." The language of "advisory," however, has important implications for the community-based nature of these groups. For example, this term may imply that community members are there simply to advise local professionals and planners or provide input. Conversely, the language of advisory could refer to residents meeting merely to be briefed on important local health issues occurring in their community. In either scenario, community members are not portrayed as having active roles in bringing about change in local health outcomes. For these reasons, the language of "health committee" may be more substantial and reflect the important role that local community members can play when organized around shared concerns or interests. In this sense, careful attention should be paid to the names of groups and reflect the community-based nature of these bodies.

Conclusion

This chapter has sought to both take stock of existing health advisory boards around the United States and provide readers with broad theoretical strokes for understanding the basic features and principles of boards, if they are to be genuinely of, by, and for communities. Also discussed are potential best practices to ensure that boards are collaborative, open, dynamic, and sensitive to cultural and democratic norms. At the same time, as these findings suggest, several different models are available for establishing community boards, and a great diversity exists in organizational, procedural, and logistical details. This study provides a snapshot of an institution of great promise that can be tailored for specific community needs and preferences.

Of course, as readers have likely gathered, this chapter is intended to provide a broad framework, while attending to specifics as they arose during data collection. As such, there are some limitations to this approach, which arose out of a web-based search of boards around the United States, filtered by certain keywords that are presumed to capture a range of institutions that serve as health advisory boards but may be called something else. As a result, some organizations with a web presence may not have been captured by this analysis, but also those organizations without a web presence – very possible considering the budgets, personnel, and origins of community-based organizations – are not represented. Nonetheless, this web-based approach provides reasonable access to the prevalence and variety of community-based citizen health organizations.

These data suggest that health advisory boards are popular tools around the country for mobilizing communities for better health. At the same time, the considerable diversity – in frequency of meetings, formal organization and rules, advertising, and governance – suggests that the purpose of health advisory boards is still being debated. The widespread recognition of their value, however, and the proliferation of attempts to form and maintain them, does indicate that health advisory boards are widely seen, if only as an aspiration, as part of the future of community-based health. In other words, if community-based projects rely on regular communication and collaboration between professionals and lay residents, groups such as health advisory boards or health committees may play an important role in increasing community participation in future health interventions.

Acknowledgments The authors gratefully acknowledge financial support from the Rural and Underserved Scholars Program at Ohio University's Heritage College of Osteopathic Medicine, with particular appreciation to Dr. Randy Longenecker, Dr. Sharon Casapulla, and Dawn Mollica, and research support from Dr. Dan Skinner.

References

Blumhagen, D. (1980). Hyper-tension: A folk illness with a medical name. *Culture, Medicine, and Psychiatry, 4*(3), 197–227.

Butterfoss, F. D. (2007). *Coalitions and partnerships in community health*. San Francisco: Jossey-Bass.

Cheah, P. Y., Lwin, K. M., Phaiphun, L., Maelankiri, L., Parker, M., Day, N. P., White, N. J., & Nostena, F. (2010). Community engagement on the Thai–Burmese border: Rationale, experience and lessons learnt. *International Health, 2*(2), 123–129.

Cornwall, A., & Jewkes, R. (1995). What is participatory research? *Social Science and Medicine, 41*(12), 1667–1676.

Encandela, J. A. (1993). Social science and the study of pain since Zborowski: A need for a new agenda. *Social Science and Medicine, 36*(6), 783–791.

Franz, B., Skinner, D., & Murphy, J. W. (2016). Changing medical relationships after the ACA: Transforming perspectives for population health. *SSM-Population Health.* dx.doi.org/10.1016/j.ssmph.2016.10.015

Friedman, M. S. (1992). *Dialogue and the human image: Beyond humanistic psychology.* New York: Sage.

Galea, S., Factor, S. H., Bonner, S., Foley, M., Freudenberg, N., Latka, M., Palermo, A. G., & Vlahov, D. (2001). Collaboration among community members, local health service providers, and researchers in an urban research center in Harlem, New York. *Public Health Reports, 116*(6), 530–539.

Holden, K., Akintobi, T., Hopkins, J., Belton, A., McGregor, B., Blanks, S., & Wrenn, G. (2016). Community engaged leadership to advance health equity and build healthier communities. *Social Sciences, 5*(1), 2.

Lwin, K., Peto, T., White, N., Day, N., Nosten, F., Parker, M., & Cheah, P. (2013). The practicality and sustainability of a community advisory board at a large medical research unit on the Thai-Myanmar border. *Health, 5,* 229–236.

Minkler, M., & Wallerstein, N. (2008). *Community-based participatory research for health: From process to outcomes.* San Francisco: Jossey-Bass.

Murphy, J. W., Franz, B. A., & Callaghan, K. A. (2016). Group maturity in a community-based project. *Social Work in Public Health, 31*(5), 341–347.

Mwinga, A., & Moodley, K. (2015). Engaging with Community Advisory Boards (CABs) in Lusaka Zambia: Perspectives from the research team and CAB members. *BMC Medical Ethics, 16,* 39.

Newman, S. D., Andrews, J. O., Magwood, G. S., Jenkins, C., Cox, M. J., & Williamson, D. C. (2011). Community advisory boards in community-based participatory research: A synthesis of best processes. *Preventing Chronic Disease, 8*(3), A70.

Orfaly, R. A., Frances, J. C., Campbell, P., Wittemore, B., Jolly, B., & Koh, H. (2005). Train-the-trainer as an educational model in public health preparedness. *Journal of Public Health Management and Practice,* Supplement, S123–S127. 2.

Pelzang, R. (2010). Time to learn: Understanding patient-centered care. *British Journal of Nursing, 19*(14), 912–917.

Quinn, S. C. (2004). Protecting human subjects: The role of community advisory boards. *American Journal of Public Health, 94*(6), 918–922.

Reddy, P., Buchanan, D., Sifunda, S., James, S., & Naidoo, M. B. (2010). The role of community advisory boards in health research: Divergent views in the South African experience. *Journal of Social Aspects of HIV/AIDS, 7*(3), 2–8.

Rosenthal, E. L., Brownstein, J. N., Rush, C. H., Hirsch, G. R., Willaert, A. M., Scott, J. R., Holderby, L. R., & Fox, D. J. (2010). Community health workers: Part of the solution. *Health Affairs, 29*(7), 1338–1342.

Shediac-Rizkallah, M. C., & Bone, L. R. (1998). Planning for the sustainability of community-based health programs: Conceptual frameworks and future directions for research, practice and policy. *Health Education Research, 13*(1), 87–108.

Wangalwa, G., Cudjoe, B., Wamalwa, D., Machira, Y., Ofware, P., Ndirangu, M., & Iiako, F. (2012). Effectiveness of Kenya's community health strategy in delivering community-based maternal and newborn Care in Busia County, Kenya: non-randomized pre-test post-test study. *The Pan African Medical Journal, 13*(Supp 1), 12–19.

Walsh, M. L., Rivers, D., Pinzon, M., Entrekin, N., Hite, E. M., & Baldwin, J. A. (2015). Assessment of the perceived role and function of a community advisory board in a NIH Center of excellence: Lessons learned. *Journal of Health Disparities Research and Practice, 8*(3), 100–108.

Williams, D. R., & Neighbors, H. (2001). Racism, discrimination, and hypertension: Evidence and needed research. *Ethnicity and Disease, 11*, 800–816.

Zola, I. (1966). Culture and symptoms-an analysis of patients presenting complaints. *American Sociological Review, 31*(5), 615–630.

Chapter 5
Dialogue, World Entry, and Community-Based Intervention

Jung Min Choi

Introduction

This chapter will focus on the concept of dialogue and its importance in understanding properly the often complex lifeworld of communities and its members (Berger and Luckman 1967). If not understood clearly, dialogue can simply be confused with conversation or even discussion. While conversation and discussion are necessary components of dialogue, by no means are they equal. With respect to community-based interventions and relevant healthcare delivery, dialogue must take center stage as the guiding principle in all facets. For without a rich understanding of dialogue, even the most supportive and well-meaning healthcare professionals such as physicians, nurses, and health promoters may engage in interventions that may be irrelevant and thus ineffective. In fact, in the absence of dialogue, communities become vulnerable to what Paulo Freire calls "cultural invasion" by experts who provide a decontextualized, or a textbook, solution that may do nothing more than reproduce, or even add to the existing problems (Freire 2009, p. 152).

This unfortunate situation is more likely to occur when experts in the field are guided by a biomedical model of health. In this model, the body is viewed as a biological machine that operates smoothly until disrupted by disease. The assumption is that the body needs a "tune-up" when equilibrium is disturbed. The problem lies within the machine (body), and the broken parts must be either fixed or replaced. Similar to how a mechanical failure is identified in an automobile, a patient goes through a series of diagnostic exams before a disease is identified, located, and treated—no fuss, no mess. In short, the biomedical model represents objectivity, reason, and efficiency.

J.M. Choi (✉)
Department Sociology, San Diego State University, San Diego, CA, USA
e-mail: jchoi@mail.sdsu.edu

Nonetheless, the biomedical model has come under attack in recent years. With the advent of narrative medicine, popularized by Rita Charon (2006), the deterministic view of disease and illness has been shown to be quite limited in the treatment of patients, especially related to chronic illness. Attention is directed almost exclusively at the body and the manifestations of the disease without problematizing why certain health risks and health conditions exist in the first place. For example, when dealing with common illnesses such as diabetes and hypertension, physicians are quick to recommend a healthier diet, exercise, and medication without taking into account the social/cultural milieu of their patients. Their recommendations simply reflect a treatment that is based on a scientific metric that is presumed to be universal. Nevertheless, while a better diet and more exercise may be helpful to patients, this recommendation may prove ineffective to certain populations.

Patients who live in poor areas may struggle to adopt this seemingly simple recommendation, not because they think that this advice is silly but because they cannot afford to follow this plan. Many people who are poor experience what is known as the "poverty penalty" where they pay more for everyday goods and services than the middle class (Caplovitz 1967; Prahalad 2004). To state clearly, poor people do not have the financial means to buy healthier foods at places like *Trader Joe's* or *Whole Foods* and join a local *24 Hour Fitness Center*. In some cases, they live in neighborhoods where any type of supermarket is nonexistent within 10 miles. These are places designated by the US Department of Agriculture as food deserts. Besides the lack of fresh and healthy foods, those who are poor often have to deal with food swamps, where high-energy and low-nutrient food stores (fast-food restaurants) disproportionally dot the community compared to supermarkets. The upshot is that even the most seemingly simple and innocuous health recommendations must include a cultural narrative if patients are to be treated properly. To borrow from C.W. Mills (1959), people must employ a "sociological imagination" where a community's biography is understood in relation to the existing socio-political milieu.

Dualism, the Rise of Objectivity, and the Scientific Method

As has been mentioned by others in this volume, communities have been understood traditionally from an objective perspective where they are viewed as distinct entities that are defined by measurable characteristics. For example, a political community is a group of disparate individuals who share a common political outlook. Individuals are free to come and go from one group to another, depending on their political palate (Goizueta 1997). Similarly, most religious communities are identified either by their type, such as Christianity or Buddhism, or by denominations, such as the Catholic Church or the United Methodist Church. And other communities are recognized through characteristics such as race, gender, and even health. The main point here is that communities have been understood as little more than the collection of discrete individuals lumped together through some shared traits (Friedman 1983).

This portrayal of community is not new. Following Rene Descartes's mind/body separation and the elevation of reason, major social theorists such as Hobbes, Locke, Comte, Durkheim, and Parsons have tended to view communities in a dualistic manner. While each employs a different social imagery, they are united by the idea that reason provides order and stability in any community. Clearly in line with dualistic thinking, each of these theorists believed that subjectivity must be pushed to the periphery if a society or community is to survive. Rather than relying on personal opinions of individuals, which are often subjective and biased, society is better served when a community employs a neutral set of standards to maintain stability (Bryant 1985). Objective facts, in other words, must be used to understand a community and act as the guiding principle in any intervention. If left up to the multiple and competing experiences and stories of individuals, communities would surely collapse. Accordingly, any characteristics that are tied to interpretation or personal experience must be superseded by objective facts that are rational.

The defining trait of dualism is the bifurcation of objectivity and subjectivity, most notably argued by Rene Descartes. Unlike his predecessors, like Plato, St. Augustine, and Thomas Aquinas, Descartes attempted to explain the order of the universe through reason rather than faith (Murphy 1989). Descartes believed that there was a rational explanation to how persons could order their lives and communities. But in order to guide society based on reason and avoid chaos, any traits associated with the *res extensa* such a emotion, personal opinion, or interpretation must be eliminated or repressed (Murphy 1989). Valid knowledge, in this sense, must not cavort with interpretation and its fickle nature. To be sure, subjectivity, personal history, or cultural values must be pushed to the periphery so that rational ideas can guide human endeavors.

Nevertheless, the obsession of unearthing empirical facts to ground society gained momentum subsequent to Descartes' demise. By the late 1600s, the idea that God was involved in ordering society became passe. Some, like Thomas Hobbes, were already suggesting that social order was a reflection of empirical causes rather than the will of God. Hobbes argues that if society is to remain stable, a valid source of empirical knowledge is necessary. For without an objective reference point, society would collapse into anarchy (Hobbes 1968). In order to curb the greed and hedonistic tendencies of human nature, argued Hobbes, a third party devoid of human emotions had to be introduced. For Hobbes, the state was the answer. As the objective third party, the state reflected an unadulterated reason. Similar to the mind/body separation initiated by Descartes (1970), Hobbes introduces his own binary vision of the world by elevating public knowledge over the private since the former is thought to be based on reason (1968). Thus, the state, which represents the epitome of public knowledge, defines the parameters of social reality. In modern parlance, expert knowledge trumps personal or community stories.

Subsequent to Hobbes, Locke argues that the state is not the proprietor of rational knowledge. Instead, rational knowledge is gained in an incremental fashion through sense impressions. The mind, then, is viewed as a *tabula rasa*, which stores pure knowledge that emanates from the world. And when enough empirical knowledge is gained through sense impressions, Locke (1956) argues, humans are able to better understand the world. Although rarely mentioned in any quantitative methodology classes in academia, Locke has been influential in opening the door to what is commonly known as "scientific methodology."

While Locke did not believe that sense impression captured pure knowledge of the world, due to the limitations of the senses, he suggests that if a better methodology can be introduced, the limitations of the senses can be mitigated and eventually overcome altogether. Clearly stated, Locke realized that human sensory organs cannot reflect properly minute particles that exist in the world. This flaw, however, does not lead to incorrect but incomplete knowledge, which can be solved quite easily through scientific progress.

With scientific rigor and proper methodological tools, Locke (1956) was certain that humans would be able to expand on existing knowledge until this base became complete. Locke believed that if the minutest particles can be observed, a firm association can be established between objects and ideas. The idea is that like an atom, if individuals could be judged objectively, then understanding communities becomes quite easy since this group is nothing more than an amalgam of these persons.

Writing against the backdrop of empiricism set out by Locke, sociologists such as Comte, Durkheim, and Parsons used various strategies to support their search for objectivity. Like his predecessors, Comte was interested in discovering *pristine* social facts that regulate human beings. He believed that social order should not depend on the arbitrariness of human thoughts but something objective. As he states, "real order of the world and reality… must always be kept in view" (Comte 1903, p. 62). And in order to capture this objective referent, Comte argued, a scientific methodology must be used so as not to distort this standard.

To be sure, social facts can be revealed only by a method unfettered by values. Accordingly, the discovery of objective truth comes through the use of well-designed scientific experiments. Comte argues that unlike the other two stages of human history (Theological and Metaphysical), the Positive Stage is distinguished by the accumulation of true knowledge through the exercise of logic and observation (Bryant 1985). Once this project is complete, human interpretations will be eclipsed by "facts." Human actions can thus be coordinated harmoniously by the knowledge gathered through science. In the end, science becomes the "great definer" of truth.

Following Comte's efforts in elevating science over metaphysical speculation with respect to social order, Durkheim introduces a biological concept to describe the complexities of a modern, industrial society. According to Durkheim (1933), a society is like a giant living organism with multiple parts that are all intricately interrelated. Just as the human body needs a brain, heart, lungs, and other major organs to guide the smooth functioning of the whole, Durkheim claims that every society has its own major organs, or institutions, that keep its stability. Similar to any organism, the goal of societies and institutions is to survive. And in order to survive, they must remain heathy and guard against any disease that may disrupt stability. But what could possibly be the agent of disruption? For Durkheim, that answer is quite simple: the human element. Durkheim (1933) believed that due to industrialization, societies were losing the social and moral fabric that once united everyone. Throughout traditional societies, mechanical solidarity ruled, where there was low division of labor and high degree of collective conscience. Stated simply, in what he called primitive societies, people generally acted and thought in a similar manner due to the homogeneous nature of the group composition. On the contrary, industrialized societies were made up of multitude of peoples, cultures, religions, and beliefs that created a low degree of social connectedness, which in turn was ripe for *anomie*. He feared that too much diversity caused a state of normlessness which left society in despair. Lacking a common moral basis, society would become pathological and thus "sick" (Durkheim 1982). In order to remedy this situation and make society healthy again, he introduces dualism. What needs to happen, suggests Durkheim, is to bifurcate the social and the individual. Because human beings are colored by their cultural and religious experiences, they cannot be objective and neutral. The parts (individuals) must be subordinate to the whole (social) if society is to survive. Channeling the ghost of John Locke, Durkheim intimates that society contains natural law that can anchor itself. Although the term "natural law" is not used by Durkheim (1973), he invokes this image when he states that "it is from society that whatever is best in us comes—all the higher forms of our behavior." And since society embodies facts, like natural law, persons should pay attention to this objective information. From Durkheim's perspective, facts are "things" (Durkheim 1982, p. 60).

In this manner, society is placed beyond human affairs. Just as Descartes claimed that the mind is divine and the body earthly, Durkheim equates society with the "sacred" while viewing the individuals as "profane." Society, being independent to the human element, serves to regulate society in an objective manner. According to Durkheim, society, through the various manifestations of empirical facts, provides an explicit referent for normative behavior. And these facts can be understood best through scientific research.

The organismic analogy put forth by Durkheim comes to fruition in Talcott Parsons' theory of structural functionalism. Stated briefly, Parsons envisions society to have various institutions linked in a structural manner. These structures are the product of social evolution. But not only are social institutions linked structurally, persons are also related in this manner through roles and role-sets. And since these roles are naturally linked, social cohesion is a by-product of persons being faithful to their respective roles. This way of understanding social relationships is known as "double contingency" (Parsons and Shils 1951, p. 16).

Furthermore, Parsons couches these role-sets within the "cybernetic hierarchy" (Jackson 1977). This scheme is characterized by a hierarchy with individuals at the bottom and "ultimate reality" at the top. The top three positions in the hierarchy—ultimate reality, social system, and cultural system—are thought to be high in information that regulates human actions. On the other hand, human beings are presumed to provide energy to keep the system functioning. In the end, the ultimate reality serves to channel properly unregulated human passion. With the help of this framework, Parsons believed that he had solved successfully the Hobbesian problem of order without reference to metaphysical abstractions.

Indeed, since Descartes' formulation of the mind/body separation, dualism has played a key role in the development of Western social science. Within this scheme, the search for objectivity involves the negation of the self. In line with Descartes' obsession to find "clear and distinct" ideas, modern social scientists seek to create a wedge between the knower and whatever is known. As a disinterested spectator, social scientists wait for the world to reveal itself. Through the manipulation of various *techne*, or technologies, researchers believe an objective reality can be preserved (Murphy 1989).

To be sure, every facet of modern social life is to be understood through the prism of science. Following this line of thinking, the ever-increasing advancement in technology is thought to improve human life, including health and healthcare delivery. Computers are used, for example, to run various models to predict behaviors of certain communities and their health outcomes without ever consulting the members of the community. The premise is that as researchers they should not get involved in the intimate aspects of a community and violate the neutrality of their expert position. Even those who do consult communities often times fail to understand fully these persons due to superficial encounters involved in traditional data collection.

The Total Market, Commodification of Health, and the Absence of Dialogue

This scenario, however, is not surprising given another dominant imagery that is in vogue today and is consistent with dualism—the "total market" (Serrano-Caldera 1995). Conjuring up the values that support the workings of the marketplace, such as individualism and competition, everyone is expected to accept a utilitarian view of the world where cost/benefit analysis is always in play. Any actions that support this model are rewarded, while deviation generates negative consequences. And why would anyone reject such values that seem natural and universal? Indeed, "individualism lies at the very core of American culture" where everyone is constantly trying to increase pleasure and decrease cost (Bellah 1985).

Rather than natural, however, individualism reflects a specific philosophy, namely, atomism. Human beings are compared to free-flowing atoms that are disconnected from one another and in need of guidance. Reminiscent of Adam Smith's "invisible hand," the market is supposed to regulate all human interactions as economic transactions. The argument is that all aspects of society are presumed to function more efficiently and effectively when individuals abide by the universal regulations of the marketplace.

But because the market presumes the scarcity of goods and services, everyone is expected to adhere to the Social Darwinian principle of the "survivor of the fittest." Communities are no exception. Following the free-market theory of Hayek (1960), defenders of neoliberalism argue that the market is beneficial for everyone since no one is left out. Persons have the opportunity to throw themselves into the fray and compete for goods and services. Healthcare is among the goods and services that is open to anyone who can pay the price. Ostensibly, the market does not discriminate based on race, gender, sexuality, or any other characteristics. The idea is that as the market expands, interconnectivity and accessibility is brought to everyone, since all persons are under the umbrella of the global market. The Durkheimian dream of having a perfect giant living organism where all parts are interconnected and interdependent free of the human element seems to be at hand through the logic of the market philosophy.

Central to this philosophy is the idea of efficiency. In order to be efficient, variations must be minimized. In this sense, diversity becomes truncated. Rather than accepting the diversity of peoples and ideas, the market favors assimilation. Since the Reagan Revolution in the early 1980s, the process of standardizing society for maximum efficiency has been driven by the neoliberal idea that "the market should be the organizing principle for all political, social, and economic decisions" (Giroux 2004, p. 2). This maxim holds true for healthcare. While many healthcare organizations appeal to the idea of patient-centered care, this is a claim that cannot be fulfilled in an environment that is driven mostly by maximizing profit margins and standardization of care. How can individuals be expected to receive personalized, relevant care when this idea violates the very logic of standardization and efficiency? And the healthcare industry's reliance on science and scientific methods, as the guiding tools for patient care, further sediments this barrier between the industry and the patients.

So once again, individuals and their needs are pushed to the periphery when the market is given the latitude to organize, supervise, and run individual lives. Just like any business organization, hospitals operate under the market rule that reflects "calculus of utility, benefit, and satisfaction against a microeconomic grid of scarcity, supply and demand, and moral value-neutrality" (Brown 2009, pp. 40–41). For example, once health is viewed to be a commodity that is bought and sold, the concept of exchange value begins to dominate the discourse in the field. Based on cost/benefit analysis, health becomes packaged as a commodity that can be sold at the highest price while incurring the lowest cost. Hospitals, then, begin to look and behave more like corporations than places that sponsor the well-being of community members. Doctors, albeit interested in treating and healing patients, must first meet the financial demands of the hospital by dealing with patients in the most efficient manner. What this scenario means is that quantity becomes more pronounced than quality of care.

Practically everyone in the United States is familiar with what is commonly called an assembly line medical practice, whereby a patient hangs around for hours in a waiting room before being ushered into an exam room, just to wait again, before meeting a doctor, who takes no more than several minutes, in total, to listen to a patient, examine, and diagnose the problem before heading out the door. To be fair, there are physicians who take more time and show sensitivity to their patients' stories and needs. But these occurrences are a rarity because this type of practice is inefficient and thus lowers the profit margin. The idea is that no one, including doctors, nurses, and receptionists, escapes the logic of the total market, which relies on a scientific metric to secure maximum profits.

The patients are thus left to "shop around" for the best deal possible among a sea of competing health organizations that include hospitals, public clinics, and private physician offices. Similar to shopping for a dress or a pair of shoes, people are responsible for buying their healthcare at a price they can afford. What is wrong with this model, ask the supporters of the market? This freedom to pick and choose creates a natural order in the healthcare industry just like any other. For example, those who can afford a multimillion dollar mansion can purchase one in Beverly Hills, CA, or Soho, NY, while those who cannot have to shop somewhere else. This principle holds true for schools, automobiles, clothing, theme parks, and restaurants. When people are able to pursue their own wants and needs based on their buying power, a natural order results (Friedman 1962). Why should health be any different?

According to Alejandro Serrano-Caldera, this world view represents a specific "ontology" that accepts competitive individualism, egocentrism, and violence as being natural. In order to succeed in this world, persons must accept assimilation. Any uniqueness related to culture, religion, ethnicity, sexual orientation, and so on must be repressed in order for the marketplace to function at the optimal level. In this regard, the world may have become more connected but not any more intimate. In the midst of incessant exchange of information via Twitter, Facebook, Snapchat, texting, and emailing, dialogue is conspicuously absent.

Dialogue and World Entry?

So, what is dialogue? According to Martin Buber, dialogue is not a conversation or a discussion between people. Likewise, dialogue is not a technique for sharing information. In fact, Martin Buber suggests that dialogue has little to do with persons speaking to each other. Obviously, conversing and discussing are a facet of interaction but they do not constitute dialogue. Instead, dialogue represents the social ontology of I and thou, that is, the fundamental practice of being in the world *together* (Buber 1958). This association involves an epistemological relationship where the other's existence is recognized entirely and fully not simply as an individual but as a community member who is always already at the table.

At this time, it is important to elaborate on the concept of "always already at the table" because this imagery is antithetical to the commonplace notion of "bringing something to the table." Unlike a community where individualism is the norm and each person is treated like an atom, in a community where dialogue is present, bringing something to the table is not a requirement to enjoy all the rights, privileges, and responsibilities of full membership. In fact, the notion of having to "bring something to the table," in this light, is quite absurd. The idea is that *everyone*, not just this or that person, has a right "to be at the table" at all times. True to the Mayan greeting, *In Lak'Ech*, every community member is viewed as the "other me."

Rather than assimilating to fit into the marketplace, dialogue presents an opening where divergent thinking and a multitude of narratives are recognized. Because the world is not a collection of disparate, objective entities but rather a patchwork of interpretive communities, a proper reading of persons or communities is paramount. To borrow from Rita Charon, communities must be understood on their own terms (Charon 2006).

But if communities have an interpretive bent and norms no longer reflect obtrusive facts, how can the norms of these groups be properly read? In the beginning this task is difficult, but not impossible. As long as people approach one another as subjects whose identities are a reflection of their life experiences and are open to reinterpretation and change, familiarity can begin to develop. But in order for this change to occur, the *lebenswelt*, or the lifeworld, of a community must be entered. But this is not an easy task since entrance into a lifeworld of a community isn't dependent on recognizing some objective empirical indicators. Instead, a person must be open to accepting the multiple layers of interpretations that emanate from the community. But if taken seriously, interpretation via world entry is the most appropriate way to understand another person or a community. Buber aptly describes this involvement as a "meeting" (Buber 1958, p. 79).

Similar to when two strangers meet for the first time, entrée into a community requires significant commitment to sharing each other's histories, while recognizing that a variety of perspectives may be operative and goals may be interpreted differently. However, through sharing and interpreting each other's viewpoints, a sense of familiarity develops. This awareness is what Schutz (1962) has in mind when he writes about "growing old" together. Each person or community must be "tuned in" to the experiential realm of the other, if proper communication is to develop.

Stability in a community is usually maintained not by following some universal standards or scientific procedures but because persons are familiar with the accepted norms and values of a particular "interpretive community" (Fish 1980, p. 14). An interpretive community, according to Stanley Fish (1989), is not merely a group of individuals who share a common interest or viewpoint but embodies the "consciousness of community members who were no longer individuals, but insofar as they were embedded in the community's enterprise, community property" (p. 141). What Fish has in mind is that since all persons are part of some interpretive community, they are not isolated atoms.

In order to have dialogue, world entry is essential. World entry involves grasping the linguistically interpreted world. Similar to an immigrant or a child, persons have to learn the various words and worlds of names, places, sounds, and so on, before a community can be understood (Lyotard 1984). To borrow from Wittgenstein (1953), all communities operate on "language games," whereby a person who enters a social situation must learn the rules that sustain the interaction that exists.

But since interpretations are based on assumptions, and assumptions tend to proliferate, a universal base of knowledge loses legitimacy. Once knowledge is understood to be formed through linguistic practices, persons no longer have to be enslaved by universal abstractions such as human nature, the state, science, or the market. And although, at times, interpretive communities may hold onto norms and values that seem to be permanent, interpretive communities are not likely to become reified. The very fact that interpretive communities reflect discursive formations based on language suggests that the permanent sedimentation of certain values is difficult.

Because world entry is at the heart of dialogue, persons must go beyond equating dialogue with concepts such as genuine discussion, engagement, understanding, transparency, or even intimacy. While all of these concepts are relevant and can elevate interpersonal connections in importance, they do not have much to do with dialogue. In the context of healthcare delivery, for example, a physician can show tremendous amount of understanding and engage a patient, and the patient may even feel a sense of intimacy with the doctor, but this sense of closeness does not mean that dialogue is present. A doctor may have the best bedside manners and yet provide a medical recommendation that violates a patient's values. Similarly, simply because doctors and patients speak the same language does not guarantee dialogue. For example, the use of translation services in hospitals frequently results in this unsavory situation where communication may be happening in the absence of dialogue. The doctor and the patient may have had an extensive discussion, but not a dialogue.

As previously mentioned, dialogue is more like a "meeting" than an encounter. According to Buber (1958), a meeting requires that persons recognize and accept the differences expressed by others (pp. 77–79). A person or community's stories must be heard and listened to, not to change or correct them but to engage in what symbolic interactionists call empathetic introspection. As Friedman (1983) notes, "only a real listening—a listening witness—can plumb the abyss of that universal existential mistrust that stands in the way of genuine dialogue and peace" (p. 258). Indeed, meetings require persons to articulate who they are as they are. Buber (1965) aptly describes this situation as follows: "[a person] can become whole not in virtue of a relation to himself but only in virtue of a relation to another self. This other self may be just as limited and conditioned as he is; in being together the unlimited and the unconditioned is experienced" (p. 168).

At this juncture is where reflection comes into play. Without reflection, dialogue is not possible. Reflection allows for a constant epistemological curiosity where persons meditate, in a critical manner, on the other's storylines. In this sense, community members can reflect not just on the concerns and desires of its members but also on the underlying assumptions that guide those concerns and desires. In this way, reflection allows persons to focus not only on symptoms but to address the root sources of a problem. The symptoms may not indicate much about a person or community; instead, they must be interpreted correctly to have any real meaning. As mentioned already, diabetes and hypertension may be symptoms of a lack of exercise or healthy diet, but the root source of these diseases may be linked to poverty—food deserts, food swamps, and the constant stress that accompanies poverty (McEwen and Lasley 2002).

Nevertheless, reflection reveals the limits and impact of storylines. Only then can persons enter into each other's lifeworld without cultural invasion where a single story dominates, intimidates, and dismisses all other narratives. Because each story has a limit and a boundary, no story can claim universality or objectivity. In this sense, even science, which is commonly associated with objectivity, reflects a particular discourse rather than the truth (Foucault 1982). Consequently, no story is viewed to be limitless or boundless, thereby the argument that one worldview is essentially or naturally superior to another loses justification.

Conclusion: Community-Based Intervention

Dialogical engagement is at the heart of this community-based philosophy. According to this perspective, researchers and the community are engaged in a committed relationship where honesty, openness, and critical conversations are not only encouraged but expected. As mentioned already, too often researchers engage in cultural invasion where they study and make decisions *on* and *for* a community without dialogue. Therefore, the needs and the desires of the community are regularly overlooked. This scenario reflects a "monological" relationship where communities are studied as "objects" by experts almost like sick "things" to be cured. The outsider (researcher) assesses a community and introduces solutions without having considered the stories of the members. This approach is a classic case of a dualistic outlook where the "expert" knowledge mutes the voice of the ordinary citizens.

At the same time, the voice of community members is not the only rudder that should steer community-based projects. This situation can result in what is known as "subjectivism" where the voices of the community are accepted without critical reflection (Freire 2009). While the experience of the community members should never be discredited or questioned, their analyses of a situation may not necessarily encompass the best possible outcome or solution to a problem.

Indeed, what is needed at this point is to eschew both the "expert" and "subjectivist" positions and adopt a strategy of "synthesis." Stated simply, synthesis requires, on the one hand, that researchers identify with a community's needs and desires and at the same time begin to view phenomena as problems in themselves! Indeed, when in a dialogical relationship, the researcher and community members are no longer severed entities who try to find a common ground. Once synthesis, or dialogue, occurs the boundaries of the researcher/community are dissolved into the "ontology of the between" (Friedman 1983). This site is where "the touchstone of reality is not the self taken by itself but the self in its relationship to other selves" (1983, p. 3). Once this transformation occurs, true community-based interventions can happen that are relevant and meaningful to communities and their members. What is left is the urgency to engage in dialogue. This process may not be easy or entirely efficient but must be done in order to bring about a world where persons live at the nexus of each other's stories—a world narrated through a tapestry of unique stories, not as experts vs ordinary citizens but as community members.

References

Bellah, R. (1985). *Habits of the heart*. Berkeley: University of California Press.
Berger, P., & Luckman, T. (1967). *The social construction of reality: A treatise in the sociology of knowledge*. Garden City: Anchor Books.
Brown, L. R. (2009). *Plan 4.0: Mobilizing to save civilization*. New York: W.W. Norton and Company.
Bryant, C. (1985). *Positivism in social theory and research*. New York: St. Martin's Press.
Buber, M. (1958). *I and thou*. New York: Charles Scribner's Sons.
Buber, M. (1965). *Between man and man*. New York: Macmillan.
Caplovitz, D. (1967). *The poor pay more: Consumer practices of low-income families*. New York: Free Press.
Charon, R. (2006). *Narrative medicine: Honoring the stories of illness*. New York: Oxford University Press.
Comte, A. (1903). *A discourse on the positive spirit*. London: William Reeves.
Descartes, R. (1970). *Discourse on method and other writings*. Middlesex: Penguin Books.
Durkheim, E. (1933). *The division of labor in society*. New York: The Free Press.
Durkheim, E. (1973). *Moral education*. New York: The Free Press.
Durkheim, E. (1982). *The rules of sociological method*. New York: The Free Press.
Fish, S. (1980). *Is there a text in this class?* Cambridge: Harvard University Press.
Fish, S. (1989). *Doing what comes naturally*. Durham: Duke University Press.
Foucault, M. (1982). *This is not a pipe*. Berkeley: University of California Press.
Freire, P. (2009). *Pedagogy of the oppressed*. New York: Continuum Books.
Friedman, M. (1962). *Capitalism and freedom*. Chicago: University of Chicago Press.
Friedman, M. (1983). *The confirmation of otherness in family, community, and society*. New York: The Pilgrim Press.
Giroux, H. (2004). *The terror of neoliberalism*. Boulder: Paradigm Publishing.
Goizueta, R. (1997). *Caminemos con Jesus: Toward a Hispanic/Latino theology of accompaniment*. New York: Orbis Books.
Hayek, F. (1960). *The constitution of liberty*. Chicago: University of Chicago Press.
Hobbes, T. (1968). *Leviathan*. New York: Penguin Books.
Jackson, T. (1977). *The evolution of societies*. Englewood Cliffs: Prentice Hall.
Locke, J. (1956). *The second treatise on government*. New York: Macmillan.
Lyotard, J. (1984). *The postmodern condition: A report on knowledge*. Minneapolis: University of Minnesota Press.
McEwen, B., & Lasley, E. (2002). *The end of stress as we know it*. New York: Dana Press.
Mills, C. W. (1959). *The sociological imagination*. London: Oxford University Press.
Murphy, J. W. (1989). *Postmodern social analysis and criticism*. Westport: Greenwood Press.
Parsons, T., & Shils, E. (1951). *Toward a general theory of action*. Cambridge: Harvard University Press.
Prahalad, C. K. (2004). *The fortune at the bottom of the pyramid*. Upper Saddle River: Wharton School Publishing.
Schutz, A. (1962). *Collected papers I: The problem of social reality*. Boston: Martinus Nijhoff.
Serrano-Caldera, A. (1995). *Los dilemmas de la democracia [The dilemmas of democracy]*. Managua: Editorial Hispamer.
Wittgenstein, L. (1953). *Philosophical investigations*. New York: Blackwell Publishing.

Chapter 6
Politics of Knowledge in Community-Based Work

Karie Jo Peralta

Introduction

There is considerable agreement that dialogue with communities is necessary to address their health concerns (Figueroa et al. 2002). Using this community-based practice (Arora et al. 2015), planners may access and navigate the interpretive realms of communities to grasp the meanings that members give to their realities (Berger and Luckmann 1967), including how they perceive their well-being, neighborhood conditions, and barriers to health care. When dialogue is sustained throughout a project (Nemeroff 2008), the opportunity is opened for every phase of an initiative to be consistent with local input, stimulated by group ideas, and motivated by the desired outcomes of a community (Eversole 2015).

Entering into dialogue requires reflexivity (Steier 1991). This process examines personal assumptions, as well as individual actions and their effects (Cunliffe and Easterby-Smith 2004). Additionally, reflexivity entails an imaginative component that helps to visualize possible ways to interact effectively with others. Reflecting is crucial in dialogue, because this act reveals the limits of perceptions shaped by past experiences, future possibilities, and beliefs of how different perspectives may merge (Husserl 1960). Influenced by Husserl (1960), Gadamer (1975) calls this blending of viewpoints a "fusion of horizons" (p. 306) that establishes common ground to achieve mutual understanding and agreement.

This level plane provides the space for different kinds of knowledge to come into view and be considered equally within a community's frame for collective interpretation. All initiatives, however, involve a variety of knowledge bases that may be incompatible with one another. So, the issue is what knowledge should shape the planning process? The purpose of this chapter is to offer insight into how

K.J. Peralta (✉)
Department of Sociology and Anthropology, University of Toledo, Toledo, OH, USA
e-mail: Karie.Peralta@utoledo.edu

community-based planners may address this question in their projects by exposing traditional assumptions and rethinking them, so that their work may be consistent with a community-based approach. At the outset, issues that preclude a community's perspective from being seen as worthy of consideration are identified. An examination of the barriers to understanding local logics is then provided, followed by a discussion of how projects may be democratized. In conclusion, the power that is released from adhering to a community-based orientation is emphasized.

Recognizing the Credibility of a Community

Hierarchy and Status

Traditional projects are designed by individuals, who are believed to hold objective viewpoints and have technical skills (Eversole 2015). Typically, these persons are "experts" or professionals, who draw conclusions about the world and its problems using a particular, fixed framework that is assumed to be applicable to all communities (Schutz 1962). Given the high level of training and education of these persons, authority is conferred commonly to them without a second thought. And, because of their high status, the ideas of planners are given significant weight, and their opinions are believed to matter most (Richard 1993).

Consequently, these persons dominate the planning process. The inclination to believe that the perspectives of planners are above critique makes their preferences appear to be naturally right for a community. Furthermore, the hidden privileges that support a planner's status make maintaining control fairly easy (Deetz 2000). By taking for granted the "abstract knowledge" (Eversole 2015, p. 92) that planners claim to be universally relevant, their positions may be imposed without much difficulty. Under these conditions, the ability for community members to take their place in dialogue is nearly impossible.

From a community-based perspective, the paternalism of traditional planning is problematic (Fals Borda 1988; Salander and Moynihan 2010), particularly when professionals approach collaborative efforts with the assumption that their stance will have a significant bearing on project goals and how objectives are to be met. Community views may thus be taken lightly, if at all. This hegemonic mode of work overlooks the possibility that community members may have different, yet possibly meaningful, positions to advance (Said 1978).

Another issue emerges when the information that specialists offer goes unquestioned by the average citizen. Such is the case when, for example, individuals accept uncritically the programs devised by public health officials, despite having doubts about their community's risk of disease. What may happen is that community members, who have a low social position, may withhold their opinions, due to feeling inferior (Freire 1970). In these situations, experts' voices and beliefs are likely to overpower interaction and be confronted with minimal contestation.

Overcoming Status Biases

Local perspectives may not be taken seriously, due to what Fricker (2007) identifies as "testimonial injustice" (p. 17), whereby prejudicial views lead to thinking that the statements, questions, and arguments made by a particular person are not deserving of attention. Simply put, a speaker's outlook is deemed to be flawed as a result of a baseless belief that the person is unreliable. The unfair judgment stems from the perception of the speaker's status. For instance, assumptions that low-income people have minimal medical knowledge may influence a physician to disregard concerns expressed by those who are poor.

An example of when this injustice may occur in a community health context is during international medical missions.[1] These short-term relief trips provide underserved communities with access to health care. During a mission, volunteer groups of First World doctors and their medical teams, with the support of local coordinators, offer basic primary care or, in some cases, more complex treatments such as surgery and therapy (for an example, see Utsey and Graham 2001). Additionally, they may donate medical supplies and facilitate learning opportunities that are intended to promote sustainable community health and well-being. Because these initiatives involve cooperation with nongovernmental organizations and address local issues, such as a lack of resources at a health clinic, they are often viewed by the volunteers to be a way to help communities (Withers et al. 2013).

Without a community-based orientation, however, mission teams may believe a community's poor health status is due to moral and/or cultural shortcomings. This "deficit thinking" (Valencia 1997, p. 2) may lead individuals to conclude that community members are unable to supply guidance on projects, even if the goal is for them to take control of their health. Thus, local views that are necessary for a community-based endeavor to thrive may be marginalized or ignored. As a result, a mission may distract, rather than strengthen, a grassroots effort.

In light of this potential problem, community-based planners should keep in mind the "humanness" (Mannheim 1956, p. 176) of participants, which means that they are always capable of contributing to an endeavor. Accordingly, they are charged with ensuring that what is said in discussion, rather than who is doing the talking, is the focus of planning (Deetz 2008). This way, the level of consideration given to ideas may not be influenced by perceptions of an individual's status (Carel and Kidd 2014). Fulfilling this responsibility involves promoting engagement that is centered on lived realities and experiential worlds, which participants linguistically determine, albeit in an incomplete way, using the terms that they contribute to the conversation (Deetz 2008).

Through engagement, ordinary community members, therefore, may be relied upon for their insight. After all, they have in-depth knowledge of their community and the capacity to come up with local solutions. Community members can also

---

[1] This example is informed by the author's experiences of participating in several medical missions in the Dominican Republic.

provide access to their realities upon which a project should be based (Gómez and Sordé Marti 2012). However, because a community-based perspective does not accept knowledge claims that assert a single truth, even their ideas should be subject to critique (Deetz 2008).

An initial step in fostering engagement is recognizing a community's credibility. From the outset, the possibility is opened for the goals of a community to fill the agenda of an intervention. The next section discusses a second step in this endeavor, that is, grasping knowledge about local realities and communal life. Without this understanding, strategies intended to integrate community members and their insight into the planning process will likely fall short of meeting their aim.

Appreciating Local Ways of Knowing

Significance Given to Lived Experience

A participatory epistemology guides community-based work (Fals Borda 1988). The key assumption is that persons are always tied to knowledge (Schwandt 1994). This belief has profound implications for how a community and its concerns are understood. Mainly, a community and its issues are not considered objectively (Cohen 1985).

Without theoretical sensitivity, the idea that community-based project planning does not involve objective perception may seem implausible or even plain wrong. After all, mainstream socialization and traditional education have taught historically the importance of deductive styles of knowing to acquire reliable and firm insight (Kwa 2011). Information that is "objective" is thus thought commonly to be not only useful, but necessary, in solving social problems.

Overcoming the challenges of a community, however, requires a theoretical shift from this dominant perspective that is grounded in "first philosophy" (Lévinas 1969), which presumes that unbiased information is located in a domain isolated from human influence. The new orientation that is community-based (Murphy 2014) recognizes how a separation between objective and subjective elements is not possible (Bordo 1987). From this outlook, information is not believed to be value-free. Rather, the interpretive element of local knowledge is appreciated (Fals Borda 1988).

This position is based on a phenomenological understanding of the meanings that persons give to their lived experiences and their community's social dynamics, culture, and history (Berger and Luckmann 1967). With an emphasis on persons' participation in the production of knowledge, attention is given to the role of human action in the creation of social worlds and their interpretations (Horkheimer 1992). Community-based planners, therefore, engage how community members make sense of their realities.

This task involves entering a community's "lifeworld" (Shutz and Luckmann 1973), that is, the negotiated principles, beliefs, and commitments that bond a group. The point is to grasp the "biography" (Berger and Luckmann 1967) of a community, which is the merging of meanings given to the members' history, traditions, norms, and interests. These biographical elements are socially constructed through discourse and human praxis and, therefore, language is particularly important for understanding how communal realities are shaped (Wittgenstein 1958).

Consistent with the "linguistic turn" (Lyotard 1984) in social philosophy, a community-based perspective recognizes that everything is known indirectly through speech. Moreover, language invents and forms, rather than reflects, reality. This crucial role that language plays in creating everyday experience means that "communicative competence" (Habermas 1970b, p. 367) is necessary to properly understand communal life and the various viewpoints that community members have about their circumstances. What this competence facilitates is entrance into the lifeworld of a community, which, in turn, allows for mutual understanding and the intersubjective, coproduction of knowledge (Gergen 2009).

The Legitimacy of Local Knowledge

An aim of community-based planning is to bring to the forefront what Foucault (1980) calls "popular knowledge" (p. 82), which refers to information that stems from the daily lives and regular routines of community members and is thus specific to a particular group. This knowledge is considered to be valuable by community-based planners (Israel et al. 1998) but has been viewed commonly to be unscientific and, therefore, deficient (Foucault 1980). The assumption is that knowledge that is scientific should be highly regarded, because of its presumed objective, neutral, and universal qualities (Schwandt 1994). Science is elevated, therefore, to a privileged status in the hierarchy of knowledge. By being established and evaluated according to principles that are grounded in realism (Durkheim 1983; Popper 1972), scientific knowledge is widely accepted and, in fact, viewed to be indisputable.

This belief is supported by the use of research practices that are guided by positivism (Delanty 1997), because they are expected to be impartial. Moreover, the way scientific knowledge is arranged and presented, for example, through graphs and charts, gives the impression that the information is precise and value-free. The "language of science" (Fischer 2000, p. 18), in particular, reinforces the idea that this kind of knowledge is superior to all others. And, when the assumption is that individuals are unable to comprehend the technical aspects of projects, because they lack familiarity with scientific terminology, important information may be withheld from a group (Forester 1980). Consequently, these persons may be marginalized from conversations that are relevant to their lives (Pedroni 2006).

The point of using a community-based approach, however, is to encourage the participation of all persons, who may be affected by an intervention (Minkler and Wallerstein 2005). Project leaders should thus take into consideration the interests that a community has in generating health knowledge and work with members to make sense of their social experiences, so that they may contribute to the interpretive process (Schulz et al. 2005). In this way, the "hermeneutical injustice" (Fricker 2007, p. 149) of prejudicially overlooking a community's logic may be avoided, and, in turn, popular knowledge may be appreciated.

Furthermore, conversations may be open enough to facilitate "mutually satisfying decisions" (Deetz 2000, p. 736) about group values that will guide the planning of a project (Deetz 2000). Community members may therefore hold one another accountable to adhere to the principles elevated through consensus. The following section expands on this important point of democratization that makes all participants responsible to the community and for its direction (Mannheim 1956).

Democratizing Health Projects

Dialogical Knowledge Production

Community-based planners presume that knowledge is socially constructed (Israel et al. 1998). This notion implies that what is known is coproduced through human action, negotiation, and confirmation that is intersubjective and reflexive (Delanty 2010). These processes are "always embodied, embedded in particular sociohistorical settings and communities, and intimately connected to the material factors through which they emerge" (Kuhn and Porter 2011, p. 18). In a word, they are non-dualistic, because knowing is always facilitated by language (Lyotard 1984). Understanding local realities thus entails relating with community members (Kuhn and Porter 2011).

Only through communal relations can knowledge be created dialogically (Gergen 2009). Therefore, the need to build relationships with a community cannot be overstated (Minkler and Wallerstein 2005). In typical projects, the practical side of this effort is what tends to be emphasized. For example, spending time with a community (Goldberg-Freeman et al. 2007), so that members become comfortable revealing how they may be struggling with illness, is assumed to be productive.

Nevertheless, if there is not an awareness of the theoretical underpinning of relationship building, communities are likely to be treated as mere objects (Buber 1970). As a result of this dehumanization, the dialogue necessary to coproduce knowledge will be hindered (Gergen 2009). Not even a significant focus on communication skills (Salmon 2010) is likely to foster mutual understanding in these impersonal relationships. Community-based planners, therefore, should not develop community relationships as if they were a means to an end. Rather, they should appreciate the energizing "associational life" (Block 2009, p. 85) of a community as important in its own right.

Community-Based Leadership

To grasp how knowledge may be produced dialogically, the "decentralization" (Ramnarayan 2011) of communities is important to visualize. This shift in imagery suggests that there is not a well-defined hierarchy with "top-down" communication and persons who control others (Whyte et al. 2003). Accordingly, decision-making is not carried out by an exclusive group of individuals (Locke 2003). For traditional planners, especially those who rely habitually on their way of thinking, the lack of a vertical power structure to support and implement a project may be difficult to imagine (Mannheim 1950). They may also share a widely held belief that leaders of projects must have unique traits or special styles (Block 2009).

In decentralized efforts, however, an assumption is that all persons have the capacity to learn, as well as teach others how to lead (Van Wart 2003). The time when individuals become community leaders is when they promote shared accountability and a united responsibility to contribute to the social fabric of the group (Block 2009). Participating in this way is important throughout a project. So, a community member, who offers this support, may become a leader at any point in time.

Therefore, a community-based approach appreciates how the social order evolves through "emergent coordination" (Uhl-Bien 2006, p. 668) that allows for plans to be organically created, modified, and/or transformed through conversations and negotiations at the local level. The main concern is with creating conditions, and facilitating an experience, that make cooperation possible, so that a project originates from communal participation (Block 2009). In this sense, an important task of leaders is to encourage others to work together toward realizing a community's vision (Uhl-Bien 2006). This endeavor is not necessarily straightforward, however, because groups often have a variety of outlooks and different interests. But, community-based projects are grounded in a philosophy that helps to guide decision-making when this challenge arises (Murphy 2014).

Overall, community-based leadership recognizes that local realities should be understood with regard for communal relations (Uhl-Bien 2006). The attention given to social affairs and interpersonal processes (Dachler 1992) makes apparent how a group's values and goals stem from interactions rather than from a specific person (Hosking 1988). The emphasis on relationships, however, calls into question the issue of power that may affect the self-governance of a community.

Egalitarian Spaces

The group dynamics of conventional planning may limit a community's perspective. In some circumstances, this issue may be the result of "groupthink" (Janis 1972), whereby the pressures to achieve agreement influence individuals to take a compliant stance. When this process occurs, the focus remains entirely on dominant ideas, and marginalized views are never made known. The problem is that communication, which would otherwise entice honest opinions out into the open, is hindered.

Countering this potentially stifling interaction in community-based initiatives is a dedication to the "democratization of culture" (Manheim 1956, p. 171). A core value is the preservation of an inclusive space where all interested individuals may engage in discussion without fear that social position or background will obscure ideas. This outlook facilitates the creation of conditions that are similar to those of "the ideal speech situation" (Habermas 1984, p. 25), particularly the openness to share and question in group debate. In this context, all viewpoints are carefully considered, and arguments may be raised by any competent member of the group at any time (Habermas 1984).

Moreover, what is crucial for a community-based endeavor is that sincere attention be given to the ideas of all persons, including those who are marginalized typically, in project activities (Minkler and Wallerstein 2005). The reason is that merely opening up discussions to community members does not necessarily mean that they are considered to be credible and that their viewpoints will be weighed fairly. After all, community members can likely sense when their position is not assessed fully and, as a result, may stop participating in a project.

The democratic foundation that is necessary for a project to become community-based hinges on the reflexivity of participants (Brown and Reitsma-Street 2003). Specifically, persons should recognize the boundaries of their partial perspective and the need to engage those of others to begin to understand fully a community and its problems (Gadamer 1975). This activity may transform mere discussion into dialogue (Buber 1970), in which all group members have equal positions in co-constructing communal knowledge (Richard 1993).

Given the heterogeneity of communities, there are likely to be various, and sometimes inconsistent, knowledge bases (Day 2006). A focus should thus be on promoting pluralism, so that not only different views may be interwoven in a project but that distinct ideas may be thoroughly engaged (hooks 2003). In this way, the common concern for power differentials that are always present in projects is likely to be addressed. Additionally, the "distorted communication" (Habermas 1970a, p. 205), whereby individuals think that they are reaching a shared understanding as they pursue undisclosed interests, may be blocked.

At this point, what should be evident is how community-based endeavors are based on social constructionism (Harris 2010). This theory of knowledge guides an appreciation of how consensus is achieved (Mangion 2011), so that planning may move forward. Essential to this effort are the criteria that are established by a community and used by its members to evaluate ideas and arguments (Habermas 1984). Knowledge should thus be viewed to be "an explicit social formation arrived at through value-laden social processes" (Deetz 1995, p. 136). What may be deemed to be "fact" is determined locally by community members through discourse (Lyotard 1984) according to collectively, though maybe temporarily, recognized standards (Habermas 1984). The grounding of these measures in cultural values and norms suggests that a project is likely to be culturally relevant, if the democratic process for generating communal knowledge is respected.

Given an emphasis on planning that is grassroots and intersubjective, health professionals may be concerned about how scientific knowledge may contribute to community-based projects. To be clear, scientific claims are not rejected automatically. Rather, they are viewed to be one among many possible answers (Vaillancourt Rosenau 1994). Consistent with this insight is the idea that knowledge does not have inherent value (Lyon and Chesebro 2011). Accordingly, scientific arguments may influence the direction of an endeavor, but they must first hold up to the scrutiny of a community.

Conclusion

Alevesson and Karreman (2001) note that "knowledge is not an innocent or neutral tool for accomplishing something socially valuable, but is closely related to power" (p. 1000). Without a community-based orientation, a community's power is likely to be suppressed and, therefore, its perspective may be ignored. Furthermore, a community's right to direct its own progress and make decisions that affect the group is bound to be violated. A project, therefore, may exploit a community rather than respond to its reality and address its priorities.

In a project that is truly community-based, however, a dialogical effort diminishes any dominance that may hinder the sharing of information and allows the collective outlook to remain salient throughout the process. Accordingly, social problems may be tackled in community-determined ways (Gibbons et al. 2016). Community-based planners should appreciate therefore the perspectives of community members and be committed to engaging their thoughts and opinions.

By following a community-based philosophy (Murphy 2014), project plans may be derived from dialogue rather than from methods that sustain a "grand narrative" (Lyotard 1984, p. 37) and serve particular interests. Accordingly, knowledge is "organized by categories socially approved" (Lazega 1992, p. 26) by community members, who promote plans that are culturally appropriate (June Yi et al. 2015). Essentially, a community is empowered to use its knowledge bases and practices for the benefit of the group.

When facilitating this process, community-based planners should reflect continually on how closely efforts are aligning with a community-based approach (Hacker 2013) and call attention to any adjustments needed along the way. Required in this task is constant attentiveness to how knowledge is created, understood, and disseminated and whether or not the interests of the community are honored during these processes. Their ultimate purpose is to keep discussions open (Deetz 2000), so that all possibilities may be explored and alternative pathways may be forged.

References

Alvesson, M., & Karreman, D. (2001). Odd couple: Making sense of the curious concept of knowledge management. *Journal of Management Studies, 38*(7), 995–1018.
Arora, P. G., Krumholz, L. S., Guerra, T., & Leff, S. S. (2015). Measuring community-based participatory research partnerships: The initial development of an assessment instrument. *Progress in Community Health Partnerships: Research, Education, and Action, 9*(4), 549–560.
Berger, P., & Luckmann, T. (1967). *The social construction of reality: A treatise in the sociology of knowledge*. Garden City: Anchor Books.
Block, P. (2009). *Community: The structure of belonging*. San Francisco: Berrett-Koehler Publishers.
Bordo, S. R. (1987). *The flight to objectivity: Essays on Cartesianism and culture*. Albany: State University of New York Press.
Brown, L., & Reitsma-Street, M. (2003). The values of community action research. *Canadian Social Work Review, 20*(1), 61–78.
Buber, M. (1970). *I and thou* (2nd ed.). New York: Charles Scribner's Sons.
Carel, H., & Kidd, I. J. (2014). Epistemic injustice in healthcare: A philosophical analysis. *Medicine, Health Care and Philosophy: A European Journal, 17*(4), 529–540.
Cohen, A. P. (1985). *The symbolic construction of community*. London: Routledge.
Cunliffe, A. L., & Easterby-Smith, M. (2004). From reflection to practical reflexivity: Experiential learning as lived experience. In M. Reynolds & R. Vince (Eds.), *Organizing reflection* (pp. 30–46). Burlington: Ashgate Publishing Company.
Dachler, H. P. (1992). Management and leadership as relational phenomena. In M. V. Cranach, W. Doise, & G. Mugny (Eds.), *Social representations and social bases of knowledge* (pp. 169–178). Lewiston: Hogrefe & Huber Publishers.
Day, G. (2006). *Community and everyday life*. New York: Routledge.
Deetz, S. (1995). *Transforming communication, transforming business: Building responsive and responsible workplaces*. Cresskill: Hampton.
Deetz, S. (2000). Putting the community into organizational science: Exploring the construction of knowledge claims. *Organization Science, 11*(6), 732–738.
Deetz, S. (2008). Engagement as co-generative theorizing. *Journal of Applied Communication Research, 36*(3), 289–297.
Delanty, G. (1997). *Social science: Beyond constructivism and realism*. Minneapolis: University of Minnesota Press.
Delanty, G. (2010). *Community* (2nd ed.). New York: Routledge.
Durkheim, E. (1983). *Pragmatism and sociology* (J.C. Whitehouse & J.B. Allcock, Trans.). Cambridge: Cambridge University Press.
Eversole, R. (2015). *Knowledge partnering for community development*. New York: Routledge.
Fals Borda, O. (1988). *Knowledge and people's power: Lessons with peasants in Nicaragua, Mexico and Colombia*. New York: New Horizons Press.
Figueroa, M.E., Kincaid, D.L., Rani, M., & Lewis, G. (2002). Communication for social change: an integrated model for measuring the process and its outcomes. Retrieved from http://www.communicationforsocialchange.org/pdf/socialchange.pdf
Fischer, F. (2000). *Citizens, experts, and the environments: The politics of local knowledge*. Durham: Duke University Press.
Forester, J. (1980). Critical theory and planning. *Journal of the American Planning Association, 46*, 275–286.
Foucault, M. (1980). Two lectures. In C. Gordon (Ed.), *Power/knowledge: Selected interviews and other writings 1972–1977* (pp. 78–108). New York: Pantheon Books.
Freire, P. (1970). *Pedagogy of the oppressed*. (M. B., Ramos, Trans.). New York: The Continuum International Publishing Group
Fricker, M. (2007). *Epistemic injustice: Power and the ethics of knowing*. Oxford: Oxford University Press.

Gadamer, H. G. (1975). *Truth and method* (2nd ed.) (J. Weinsheimer & D. Marshall, Trans.). New York: The Continuum Publishing Company.

Gergen, K. J. (2009). *An invitation to social construction* (2nd ed.). Thousand Oaks: Sage.

Gibbons, M. C., Illangasekare, S. L., Smith, E., & Kub, J. (2016). A community health initiative: Evaluation and early lessons learned. *Progress in Community Health Partnerships: Research, Education, and Action, 10*(1), 89–101.

Goldberg-Freman, C., Kass, N., Ross, G., Bates-Hopkins, B., Purnell, L., Canniffe, B., & Farfel, M. (2007). You've got to *understand* community: Community perceptions on "breaking the disconnect" between researchers and communities. *Progress in Community Health Partnerships: Research, Education, and Action, 1*(3), 231–240.

Gómez, A., & Sordé Marti, T. (2012). A critical communicative perspective on community research: Reflections on experiences of working with Roma in Spain. In L. Goodson & J. Phillimore (Eds.), *Community research for participation: From theory to method* (pp. 21–35). Chicago: The Policy Press.

Habermas, J. (1970a). On distorted communication. *Inquiry, 13*(1–4), 205–218.

Habermas, J. (1970b). Towards a theory of communicative competence. *Inquiry, 13*(1–4), 360–375.

Habermas, J. (1984). *Theory of communicative action, Vol 1: Reason and the rationalization of society* (T. McCarthy, Trans.). Boston: Beacon Press.

Hacker, K. (2013). *Community-based participatory research*. New York: SAGE Publications.

Harris, S. R. (2010). *What is constructionism? Navigating its use in sociology*. Boulder: Lynne Rienner Publishers.

Hooks, b. (2003). *Teaching community: A pedagogy of hope*. New York: Routledge.

Horkheimer, M. (1992). Traditional and critical theory. In D. Ingram & J. Simon-Ingram (Eds.), *Critical theory: The essential readings* (pp. 239–254). New York: Paragon House.

Hosking, D. M. (1988). Organizing, leadership, and skillful process. *Journal of Management Studies, 25*, 147–166.

Husserl, E. (1960). *Cartesian meditations: An introduction to phenomenology* (D. Cairns, Trans.). The Hague: Martinus Nijhoff.

Israel, B. A., Schulz, A. J., Parker, E. A., & Becker, A. B. (1998). Review of community-based research: Assessing partnership approaches to improve public health. *Annual Review of Public Health, 19*, 173–202.

Janis, I. L. (1972). *Victims of groupthink*. Boston: Houghton Mifflin.

June Yi, K., Landais, E., Kolahdooz, F., & Sharma, S. (2015). Framing health matters: Factors influencing the health and wellness of urban aboriginal youths in Canada: Insights of in-service professionals, care providers, and stakeholders. *American Journal of Public Health, 105*(5), 881–890.

Kuhn, T., & Porter, A. J. (2011). Heterogeneity in knowledge and knowing: A social practice perspective. In H. E. Canary & R. D. McPhee (Eds.), *Communication and organizational knowledge: Contemporary issues for theory and practice* (pp. 17–34). New York: Routledge.

Kwa, C. (2011). *Styles of knowing: A new history of science from ancient times to the present* (D. McKay, Trans.). Pittsburgh: University of Pittsburgh Press.

Lazega, E. (1992). *Micropolitics of knowledge: Communication and indirect control in work groups*. New York: Aldine de Gruyter.

Lévinas, E. (1969). *Totality and infinity*. Pittsburgh: Duquesne University Press.

Locke, E. A. (2003). Leadership: Starting at the top. In C. L. Pearce & J. A. Conger (Eds.), *Shared leadership: Reframing the hows and whys of leadership* (pp. 271–284). Thousand Oaks: Sage.

Lyon, A., & Chesebro, J. L. (2011). The politics of knowledge: A critical perspective on organizational knowledge. In H. E. Canary & R. D. McPhee (Eds.), *Communication and organizational knowledge: Contemporary issues for theory and practice* (pp. 69–86). New York: Routledge.

Lyotard, J. (1984). *The postmodern condition*. Minneapolis: University of Minnesota Press.

Mangion, C. (2011). *Philosophical approaches to communication*. Bristol: Intellect.

Mannheim, K. (1950). *Freedom, power, and democratic planning*. London: Oxford University Press.

Mannheim, K. (1956). *Essays on the sociology of culture: Collected works of Karl Mannheim* (Vol. 7). New York: Routledge.

Minkler, M., & Wallerstein, N. (2005). Improving health through community organization and community building: A health education perspective. In M. Minkler (Ed.), *Community organizing and community building for health* (2nd ed., pp. 26–50). New Brunswick: Rutgers University Press.

Murphy, J. W. (2014). *Community-based interventions: Philosophy and action.* New York: Springer.

Nemeroff, T. (2008). Generating the power for development through sustained dialogue: An experience from rural South Africa. *Action Research, 6*(2), 213–232.

Pedroni, T. C. (2006). Can the subaltern act? African American involvement in educational voucher plans. In M. W. Apple & K. L. Buras (Eds.), *The subaltern speak: Curriculum, power, and educational struggles* (pp. 95–117). New York: Routledge.

Popper, K. (1972). *The logic of scientific discovery.* London: Hutchinson.

Ramnarayan, S. (2011). Participation: Considerations for designing process. In S. Ramnarayan & T. V. Rao (Eds.), *Organization development: Accelerating learning and transformation* (2nd ed., pp. 267–276). Thousand Oaks: Sage.

Richard, N. (1993). Postmodernism and periphery. In T. Docherty (Ed.), *Postmodernism: A reader* (pp. 463–470). New York: Columbia University Press.

Said, E. W. (1978). *Orientalism.* New York: Pantheon.

Salander, P., & Moynihan, C. (2010). Facilitating patients' hope work through relationship: A critique of the discourse of autonomy. In R. Harris, N. Wathen, & S. Wyatt (Eds.), *Configuring health consumers: Health work and the imperative of personal responsibility* (pp. 113–125). New York: Palgrave Macmillan.

Salmon, P. (2010). The work of clinical communication in cancer care. In R. Harris, N. Wathen, & S. Wyatt (Eds.), *Configuring health consumers: Health work and the imperative of personal responsibility* (pp. 126–139). New York: Palgrave Macmillan.

Schulz, A. J., Zenk, S., Odoms-Young, A., Hollis-Neely, T., Nwankwo, R., Lockett, M., et al. (2005). Healthy eating and exercising to reduce diabetes: Exploring the potential of social determinants of health frameworks within the context of community-based participatory diabetes prevention. *American Journal of Public Health, 95*(4), 645–651.

Schutz, A. (1962). *Collected papers I: The problem of social reality.* The Hague: Martinus Nijhoff.

Schutz, A., & Luckmann, T. (1973). *The structure of the life-world (vol. 1)* (R. M. Zaner & H. T. Engelhardt, Jr., Trans.). Evanston: Northwestern University Press.

Schwandt, T. A. (1994). Constructivist, interpretivist approaches to human inquiry. In N. K. Denzin & Y. S. Lincoln (Eds.), *Handbook of qualitative research* (pp. 118–137). Thousand Oaks: Sage.

Steier, F. (1991). Introduction: Research as self-reflexivity, self-reflexivity as social process. In F. Steier (Ed.), *Research and reflexivity* (pp. 1–11). Newbury Park: Sage.

Uhl-Bien, M. (2006). *Relational leadership theory: Exploring the social processes of leadership and organizing.* Leadership Institute Faculty Publications. Paper 19. Retrieved from https://pdfs.semanticscholar.org/e77e/af0079f4c66c03eaddfb71bc181fbd0d28a5.pdf

Utsey, C., & Graham, C. (2001). Investigation of interdisciplinary learning by physical therapist students during a community-based medical mission trip. *Journal of Physical Therapy Education, 15*(1), 53–59.

Vaillancourt Rosenau, P. (1994). Health politics meets post-modernism: Its meaning and implications for community health organizing. *Journal of Health Politics, Policy and Law, 19*(2), 303–333.

Valencia, R. R. (1997). Conceptualizing the notion of deficit thinking. In R. R. Valencia (Ed.), *The evolution of deficit thinking: Educational thought and practice.* Oxon: RoutledgeFalmer.

Van Wart, M. (2003). Public-sector leadership theory: An assessment. *Public Administration Review, 63*(2), 214–228.

Whyte, W. F., Blasi, J. R., & Kruse, D. L. (2003). Worker ownership, participation and control: Toward a theoretical model. In M. J. Handel (Ed.), *The sociology of organizations: Classic, contemporary, and critical readings* (pp. 475–501). Thousand Oaks: Sage Publications.

Withers, M., Browner, C. H., & Aghaloo, T. (2013). Promoting volunteerism in global health: Lessons from a medical mission in northern Mexico. *Journal of Community Health, 38*(2), 374–384.

Wittgenstein, L. (1958). *The blue and brown books.* New York: Harper and Row.

Chapter 7
Community Mapping Tells an Important Story

Karen A. Callaghan

Introduction

The Alma-Ata (1978) and Ottawa (1986) conferences, sponsored by the World Health Organization (WHO), are considered watershed moments in the primary health-care movement. Since 1978, governments, medical professionals, and other practitioners have been challenged to provide "Health for All." This simple slogan represents profound shifts in assumptions about health, illness, delivery modalities, and the relationships and status of patients and care providers. Succinctly, health care for all is considered possible only through a holistic view of health and a participatory, community-based orientation. Furthermore, poor health is considered to be the outcome of policies and practices that create unequal access to care and basic resources (Kickbusch 2003).

The Alma-Ata Declaration (1978) equates health with "complete mental, physical, and social well-being, and not merely the absence of disease or infirmity." Hence, in order to achieve good health, persons' relationships, employment, living environment, educational opportunities, and overall development must be well-functioning and satisfying. Individual physiological states can no longer be understood in isolation from the social context of everyday life. The quality of one's social network, as well as access to needed resources, corresponds to overall health status and outcomes.

Within this framework, the focus of the health-care system must shift from treatment of disease to prevention and health promotion. Accordingly, effective care must address the myriad complex issues related to physical and social well-being. Health promotion must be democratic, since the process for creating well-being is driven by communities working collaboratively with various practitioners,

K.A. Callaghan (✉)
Department of Sociology and Criminology, Barry University, Miami, FL, USA
e-mail: kcallaghan@barry.edu

policy makers, planning organizations, and government agencies (WHO 1986). Health-care providers are concerned, then, with what the traditional biomedical model would classify as social and political issues. Health promotion and intervention strategies require maximizing not only access to care and treatment but ensuring direct community participation in needs and assets identification, planning, advocacy, and policy making.

Numerous strategies and approaches have been launched to address this reconceptualization of health and health care. The field of public health was dramatically impacted by the WHO initiatives, which led to calls for reorienting health service delivery, particularly to poor and underserved communities (Greco et al. 2016). These "new public health" practices, consequently, require social and political action that would lead to persons and communities having increased control of their health and health care (Awofeso 2004).

The WHO European Healthy Cities project is an example of a new public health initiative, which stipulates that urban planning projects and policies are expected to comprehensively address equity issues, the social, cultural, and environmental determinants of health, and local involvement and empowerment (de Leeuw 2011). This "healthy urban planning" approach is based on a number of key indicators, such as the quality and accessibility of housing, water, sanitation, food, employment opportunities, social networks, and basic services and facilities (education, recreation, health care) (de Leeuw et al. 2015). In addition, local government agencies, planning boards, and advocacy and direct service organizations are expected to work collaboratively and be held accountable for developing and sustaining healthy living environments (Barton and Grant 2011).

The field of social epidemiology has generated more multidimensional, non-reductionist explanations of health and disease distribution and prevention. As Nancy Krieger (2001) contends, an eco-social framework for understanding the interplay between biological conditions and the social reproduction of inequalities is necessary. Epidemiological studies should address not only unequal access to good quality health care but also institutional and structural oppression and privilege, aggressive marketing of unhealthy products and lifestyles, and the stress caused by social inequalities (Krieger 2009). Hence, the sociopolitical context of attaining and maintaining health and the experience of living as part of an oppressed, excluded community are key factors to be considered for any valid epidemiological analysis.

Popular epidemiology emerged as an approach that directly addresses the role of residents, activists, and other "lay" persons in the discovery, investigation, and eradication of the illness and disease. Brown (1997) refers to this approach as both a "citizen science" and a social movement, where scientific methodologies are partnered with more subjective but equally valid ways of knowing and discernment (p. 137). This framework supports direct activist and community partnerships with scientists and other practitioners, as well as lay persons conducting formal and informal health studies.

More recently, the terms population health and population medicine have been used to focus attention on the numerous individual and systemic variables (income, physical environment, personal choices, physiology, and available services) that impact health and health outcomes. While this maneuver may seem redundant considering the new public health movement, concerns have been raised that public health efforts, particularly in the United States, are limited to specific government-sponsored programming. Public health workers, according to this analysis, are often curtailed from affecting changes in the educational, economic, and political institutions that play such an important role in creating healthy environments (Kindig and Stoddart 2003).

The introduction of these new terms is intended to point to a broader interface of researchers, policy makers, resource allocation agencies, and medical practitioners in understanding the multiple determinants of health across different populations (Kindig 2007). Nonetheless, the advances in the new public health and epidemiological fields have gained minimal status in the professional medical community (Gary and Ricciardi 2010). Clinical care remains typically focused on the diagnosis and treatment of the individual patient. Hence, the notion of population medicine is an attempt to legitimize efforts of the *medical* care system to understand and promote health beyond the direct treatment setting.

An ongoing concern with all of these approaches is the extent to which direct community participation is supported as a human right, as well as *the* integral component to developing authentic knowledge of the social and environmental context of health and health promotion. However, identifying social, economic, and political issues as legitimate topics for public health and epidemiological studies is not the same thing as promoting direct community involvement and control. While more holistic models of health that address, for example, poverty, racism, toxic environments, and exploitative working conditions, are preferable to one-dimensional clinical approaches, the actual communities in question are usually excluded from engaging as legitimate participants in analysis, decision-making, and planning. This exclusion may take the form of either the complete absence of community members or the tokenism of adding one or two representatives to advisory boards or committees.

Community-based approaches have been adopted to facilitate more in-depth involvement and collaborative partnerships between residents and various practitioners. However, in order to fully implement a community-based model, an important contradiction must be resolved. The traditional biomedical science-based approach to health and illness precludes, or at least seriously diminishes, the involvement of non-experts and the use of what is considered "subjective" information and analysis. This perspective relies, obviously, on the notion that health and other needs should be addressed by professional experts who can diagnose problems and develop remedies in isolation from "target populations." When expertise is viewed as knowledge derived from privileged sources, communities are cast as objects to be manipulated, as locations of problematized events and conditions.

In fact, within this framework, intimate or even immediate contact with persons is viewed as possibly tainting the objectivity and "cold analysis" that will lead to the desired outcomes. Any community involvement, if necessary, must be regimented according to accepted research and treatment protocols; otherwise, the information or data gathered is viewed as too subjective, that is, shaped by values, opinions, and beliefs. Within these parameters, a community cannot produce or analyze knowledge. Only those agencies and researchers with the appropriate technical expertise can deploy rigorous collection methods and extract reliable, valid data from and about a community. Information that does not meet these standards is deemed untrustworthy and irrelevant.

Even more qualitative methodologies can preclude authentic community participation. These approaches usually rely on the identification of key informants or gatekeepers within a community. Focus groups are used also to gather multiple perspectives on particular issues or problems. The viewpoints of these "strategic" persons are elevated in importance and seen as providing insights that everyday community members may not possess. More important, while these approaches often appear to be participatory, an extraction orientation may still be at work. The collection, analysis, interpretation, and use of the information remain in the hands of professional researchers, planners, and service providers. Hence, the community under scrutiny becomes only a facsimile; the actual persons involved are replaced by objective referents to problems, locations, and outcomes.

Community-based approaches would be able to facilitate more democratic participation that leads to legitimate decision-making and control only if a crucial epistemological shift occurs. This shift requires moving away from the dualism that supports the biomedical-scientific paradigm and the distinction between objectivity and subjectivity. Such a maneuver allows for an alternative understanding of how knowledge, community, and human action are constituted: a strategy that can sustain authentic inclusiveness of multiple perspectives, experiences, and interpretations (Fals Borda 2013).

Community-Based Philosophy: Narratives and Dialogue

Within the framework of an anti-dualistic philosophy, all knowledge, even an objective "fact," is derived from particular perspectives or interpretations (Murphy 2014). Professional expertise about health and health promotion is, likewise, one particular form of conceptualizing and interpreting a situation. These approaches may contain useful information and practices, but the relevance and validity for any community cannot be assumed. In other words, the validity of any knowledge cannot be demonstrated via a methodological framework. The "reality" of community life, health, or well-being cannot be grasped through an analysis of the correlations among various social indictors or other empirical referents. These elements may appear to point to significant attributes that help define and shape a community. However, little is revealed about the experiences and interpretations of the actual persons under scrutiny. These "lived experiences" cannot be portrayed adequately as another piece of data added to a logic model of decision-making and problem-solving.

When dualism is jettisoned, the focus for practitioners and researchers is shifted from extracting data to gaining entrée to a lived social world. A community, in this framework, is constituted by personal and collective interpretations, perspectives, standpoints, values, and definitions. The order or organization of a community is likewise constructed or negotiated. This order, however, is not static or monolithic and may be fraught with conflict and strife. Nonetheless, from a constructionist perspective, all social organization is derived from human action or agency.

As Berger and Luckman (1966) suggest, a community is a lifeworld or a complex of meaning, which is continually interpreted and reinterpreted as persons engage with others and try to make sense of their everyday lives (pp. 64–65). Human agency is evident in all facets of experience. Persons' lives and their situations are not passive manifestations of underlying social, physical, or psychological factors nor are they merely responses to events or circumstances. Regardless of the lack of resources and difficulties faced, persons construct meaningful interpretations of their lives and act and interact accordingly. Hence, as phenomenologists have claimed, human action is always intentional, i.e., always makes sense according to a particular perspective or set of experiences (Berger and Luckman 1966, pp. 20–21).

A community-based approach then must begin with the premise that communities have biographies (Murphy 2014, pp. 25–26). To understand how health and well-being might be maintained, the stories or narratives of how communities define and navigate these conditions must be understood. Biographical or local knowledge, rather than statistical indicators, is the most crucial component of planning, research, and intervention. The process for community participation, based on this approach, must allow multiple narratives, plots, and characters to be revealed. As with any biography, readers must be open to receiving the story, which may be inspiring, tragic, heroic, or just plain ordinary. Regardless of the tone, all stories have an internal coherence, history, highlights, and numerous characters and, most important, are told from a complex of standpoints or perspectives. Furthermore, a community cannot be reduced to a singular biography. Multiple layers of reality that often are contradictory and confusing must be assumed. Gaining entrée to a community must begin then with listening and dialogue.

However, grasping the lived experiences and interpretations of a community is not simply a technical process. Most researchers and practitioners probably assume that they listen to their subjects or patients. However, transferring information and data from one location to another is not the same thing as listening. Likewise, employing a type of cultural competence in order to ensure acceptance and compliance with planning, research, or treatment procedures is not equivalent to entering and being accepted as part of a community's social world. While communicating in relevant language, not violating social norms, and visiting persons' homes may appear to be community-based, such practices may still be paternalistic. Perhaps most important, true dialogue cannot be established without critical reflection on the distinction between local and expert knowledge.

An authentic dialogue can be established only when local narratives are taken seriously as legitimate knowledge developed about and by the community (Fals Borda 2013, p. 160). Furthermore, expert knowledge must be considered another type of narrative, developed by professional communities as they attempt to solve human and social problems. Professionals can begin to gain entrée to a community only with a sense of humility and genuine interest in learning. As Schutz (1967) notes, a researcher or practitioner is "still a human being among other human beings" (p. 221). Hence, intimate relationships can be formed to allow stories to be revealed and affirmed. Affirming community narratives does not mean simply taking note of all the details of a case history. After all, narratives reveal the complex of meaning and the interpretations and perspectives persons and communities have constructed. These stories, accordingly, should not be distilled into case notes or survey responses. On the other hand, narratives are affirmed when the world is grasped or understood genuinely from the standpoint or perspective of a community. But sustained democratic relationships among residents, researchers, and practitioners must be formed in order for community participation and control to be realized.

Hence, a true dialogue ensues when local knowledge is considered a legitimate standpoint for making sense of the world. At this point, community residents and professionals are able to begin to co-constitute interventions, planning, and further investigations. The point of dialogue is for all parties to engage in critical self-reflection, so that all narratives, with their limitations and possibilities, can provide a context for understanding and action. Once researchers and practitioners have established dialogical relationships with community residents, the possibility of various interventions or changes can be explored democratically.

Community-Based Participatory Research: Empowerment

Participatory action research methodologies provide a variety of strategies for communities to coproduce investigations, planning, and interventions. This approach is influenced by the work of Paulo Freire (1992) and Orlando Fals Borda (1988). For both writers, traditional means of teaching and research inevitably lead to a decontextualized understanding of how persons and communities exist. Furthermore, the world views or standpoints of others in more privileged positions are usually superimposed on impoverished and disenfranchised communities.

The point of teaching and research, therefore, must be empowerment. But within an anti-dualistic framework, empowerment does not mean that professional experts arrive to bestow information, resources, or control on communities. Communities already have the power to be self-governing and self-sustaining and may be engaged actively in resisting exploitive policies and practices. However, researchers and practitioners can assist communities with developing what Charles Kieffer (1984) called more effective "participatory competence" (p. 18). This process must involve open dialogue as communities are presented with different ways of interpreting situations, problems, strategies, and skills. When a democratic space has been created, communities are then able to decide if the perspectives and methods of the researcher or practitioner are relevant and useful (Solomon 1976, p. 26).

The dynamics of research, social and health planning, and other professional practices change dramatically within this framework. Specifically, professionals must find ways to engage intimately and develop trust with communities. They must understand and accept community narratives on their own terms and then share their knowledge and skills as viable alternatives for solving problems and planning interventions. Proposed research methods, questions, and instruments are reviewed and, if necessary, redesigned by community members, since they must be treated as "first among equals" in this process (Blumenthal et al. 2013, p. 7). In this framework, interpretation and analysis of research results are a collective endeavor involving discussion, debates, and final approvals from the community.

Participatory planning typically involves the formation of community-based committees, which serve as liaisons between the residents and medical, research, and policy-making professionals and institutions. In many cases, the membership of these committees is recommended or elected by local residents. These committees are responsible for organizing open channels, within the community, for communication, participation, and decision-making. Local residents learn skills for conducting needs and assets assessments, collaborating with policy makers, and participating fully in coordinating services and planning. Accordingly, participatory competence or community capacity for engaging in self-advocacy, developing political savvy and clout, and formulating plans and policies is greatly enhanced.

Community-Based Participatory Mapping: Cocreating a Social World

Neighborhood or community mapping is now a common practice in community organizing, health planning, and community development projects. For many decades community maps have been used to illustrate the spatial clustering of various social, economic, and health-related problems, along with the availability of resources and institutional support in specific neighborhoods (Sampson et al. 2002). Such mapping is considered especially useful for presenting a more holistic "picture" of community needs and assets to politicians, policy makers, and service providers. Disparities in resource allocation and access to basic services can thus be readily identified. However, in order for community mapping to become more than a "visual representation of data by geography and location," a community-based participatory philosophy and methodology must be employed (Kirschenbaum and Corburn 2012, p. 444).

From a community-based perspective, space and other physical dimensions are also lived experiences. The stories of a community reveal the ways persons interpret and produce what is considered the space where they live. Consequently, reliance on *empirical indictors* to understand spatial dimensions will result in a disembodied or abstract rendition of the community. As an empirical entity, space can be defined and measured objectively. Accordingly, health research and planning are often carried out assuming that space is neutral and can be accessed and used in a uniform and consistent manner.

In the field of medical or health geography, for example, a geographic information system (GIS) is used typically to map and match the distribution of disease with health-care providers. These studies usually rely on government census data to define specific population regions and calculate "location quotients" to determine whether rates of disease or the number of health-care providers is above or below national averages (Photis 2016, p. 3). In the end, this method of mapping allows electronic surveillance to substitute for community engagement. The community is the silent, passive recipient of aid once all important information is revealed through a map plotted with objective data.

Contrary to this methodology, in participatory community-based mapping, physical dimensions are understood to be embodied and socially constructed. As a result, space can no longer be considered neutral or empirical. Embodied dimensions are situated; their meaning and purpose are tied to personal and collection action and interaction. Distance, borders, center-periphery, and connections are defined and negotiated and do not necessarily correspond to geographic measurement. The lived experiences of residents shape what is considered near, far, or accessible.

Many health geographers, such as Hawthorne and Kwan (2011), have recognized the need for a more "contextualized" understanding of how space is experienced (p. 21). Their research on the "perceived distance" of local residents indicates that accessibility cannot be understood properly by using what are considered the "objective street network distance measures" (Hawthorne and Kwan 2011, pp. 21–22). Using this standard protocol, health planners assume that clinics and other service providers should be located within a 1 mile radius of targeted persons' homes. However, residents' "perceived distance" can be shaped by experiences such as wait time, quality of care, providers' communication skills and attitudes, and overall comfort level with the neighborhood and other clients. Hawthorne and Kwan (2011) report that residents will consider providers that are several miles from their homes to be the most accessible, that is, the "nearest" in practice, even though other facilities may exist within closer geographic proximity (p. 22).

Even those researchers who rely on GIS mapping and use census tracts and zip codes to define communities and neighborhoods often encounter what they consider to be the "subjective definitions of neighborhoods" that defy the accepted logic of using space (Campbell et al. 2009, pp. 463–464). The same business areas, high-traffic streets, and parks may be boundaries for some neighborhoods and central spots for others. Residents, for example, define "safe" spaces and street routes for their children according to recent crime events, family feuds, and gang territories. Consequently, communities do not conform to census maps or zip codes boundaries (Coulton et al. 2001, 2013). The street networks that exist, however, can be understood to make sense only from the standpoint of the communities under consideration (Coulton et al. 2011).

Mapping, then, must begin with the community and with constructing a dialogical process for revealing local knowledge. Gaining entrée can begin through local clubs, advocacy groups, churches, and other community-based organizations. However, an authentic mapping project will reveal the multiple, fluid layers of reality that exist within a community. Relying solely on the perspectives of select leaders, groups, or organizations should thus be avoided. Each of these bodies has established connections, relationships, and possibly contested interpretations with others (Elwood 2006; Blumenthal et al. 2013). They can contribute valuable information and resources to a project but should not be considered the sole authority on local knowledge.

Democratic and inclusive mapping processes are essential for understanding local debates, coalitions, and controversies. Researchers and practitioners can work with community-based organizations to create local health committees, for example, which over time become increasingly inclusive. In addition, a thorough mapping process requires creating and recreating multiple maps that can be used as tools for consensus building or reaching an intentional strategic equilibrium among community members.

Participatory mapping projects are initiated with local residents granting admission to their community by literally leading the way through a walkabout. The point of the walkabout is not simply to record the street networks of a neighborhood or to learn the location of useful services. On the contrary, this process initiates the dialogical character of a community-based project. Those who lead the walk begin to converse with other residents, introduce the project members, explain the purpose or goal of the project (if at least a tentative target issue has been identified), and invite residents to participate in the mapping process. As these conversations develop and expand, the stories of the community are told. Community members are not asked to play the role of research subjects but instead are invited to contribute their local knowledge, perspectives, viewpoints, and expertise to the mapping project. These "open air" conversations disclose the debates, connections, challenges, and disputes that constitute life in the community (Murphy et al. 2015).

After the first walkabout, plans are usually made for how the mapping process will continue and expand. Local residents can identify the most appropriate modes of communication, which often include more walkabout trips, town hall meetings, contact with established groups, block parties, and home visits. The actual mapping processes should be selected according to what resources may be available and what makes practical sense for the community and the researchers and practitioners. Maps can be hand drawn, illustrated with color photographs, and even painted on a wall or canvas. However, in order to maintain a community-based approach, the techniques used should be simple and accessible so that anyone in the community can help create maps (Chambers 2006). The point is not to recreate a predefined, objective space but to portray the lived experiences of the community. The initial mapping process is essentially a learning experience for the researchers and practitioners, as local residents provide guidance and begin to reveal the knowledge base of the community. Entrée has been accomplished when the conditions have been created to allow for more complex dialogue.

As the mapping process develops, community residents are directly involved in sharing knowledge and, importantly, in critically reflecting on the purpose and design of the project. The community situates and provides intentionally for the project. This role presents an opportunity for community members to reflect on their identities, needs, and assets as persons and as members of a collective. In the tradition of the participatory learning and action (PLA) approach, from the field of international rural land research and development, communities can engage in mapping processes that build critical consciousness and document histories of neglect and marginalization (International Fund for Agricultural Development (IFAD) 2009). Through a PLA approach, researchers and practitioners can assist communities with enhancing dispute resolution, communication, problem-solving, and organizational skills. In this regard, mapping processes can focus on community identity, aspirations, and strategies for interventions.

The initial mapping process helps communities reflect critically on an identity. From a community-based perspective, identity is not a definition that is fixed or dependent on stability, uniformity, or lack of conflict. A community's identity can be diverse or "loosely coupled" and include consensus and agreements as well as conflicts and disputes (Weick 1976). Through mapping, communities define those persons and groups who should be included in the dialogue about local issues, assets, needs, controversies, and disputes. A final consensus is not needed; effective strategies for intervention and change can be developed within a framework of multiple viewpoints, interests, and contested issues. As a democratic process, contested and controversial interpretations, alliances, and actions should be addressed as maps are collectively examined and critiqued. Dialogue about identity is facilitated by meetings devoted to comparing and discussing different versions of community maps. The issues revealed through this process may lead to creating maps based on any aspect of social identity (age, gender, religion), needs, or interests. Furthermore, the diversity of the community can be explored and acknowledged through this process.

Communities can be encouraged also to create aspirational maps, that is, to reveal a vision of community life based on persons' hopes and ideals. This process is effective in evaluating current needs and assets, in the sense that identifying aspirations requires reflection on how existing conditions should be changed and improved. This aspect of the mapping process reveals the collective efficacy (activism, resistance, organizing) and other means for mobilization within the community. A framework for intervention is created, in addition to fostering reflection on the skills, relationships, interactions, and planning that might be useful for addressing salient problems. In a large-scale mapping project in South Los Angeles, for example, a map was created to show resources for activism. A variety of local shops, churches, and gathering places that had a history of local ownership/patronage and support for community building and activism were documented with photographs (Stokes et al. 2015, pp. 62–65).

Consistent with the aim of direct community involvement and control over interventions and planning, counter-mapping is a process that can be used to develop specific campaigns or strategies for identified issues or problems. In this phase of mapping, the community develops targeted responses to official maps and other data used by government bodies, health agencies, and planning authorities. Maps plotted with objective referents to identity, needs, and problems can be challenged with experiential or narrative-based maps of community life. Rather than "ground-truthed" (geographically accurate), counter-maps can be "community-truthed" (IFAD, p. 15).

Researchers and practitioners can assist with this process by sharing their knowledge and skills, including how to collect and organize relevant information, and communicate and interact effectively with planning committees and commissions, local government agencies, service provides, and other relevant groups. Counter-mapping is a process of self-advocacy and self-determination through which communities can engage directly in shaping the official and publically accepted view of their identity and status. In the South Los Angeles project, local residents launched a media campaign to combat what they defined as "the inaccurate and fear-based image" of their community (Stokes et al. 2015, p. 57). With the assistance of university researchers, community members compiled crime statistics and a comprehensive report from a local university to demonstrate that chronic underinvestment and discrimination, rather than the conduct of residents, were the more salient obstacles to development. Maps were created and distributed to allow "outsiders" to safely visit the community, ideally as part of a bike tour. By taking the tour mapped by local residents, visitors could see the community in a different, positive context (Stokes et al. 2015, pp. 58–60).

Mapping projects can cover many other facets of community needs and aspirations. As residents are supported to create and employ different types of maps, their capacity for self-reflection, planning, organizing, and advocacy will be enhanced. Researchers and practitioners can play the role of facilitator and support system for as long as they are needed. Over time, communities can use mapping processes as a means to communicate their realities to a myriad of external agencies, service providers, and planning bodies and to stipulate that a community-based approach is mandatory for successful partnerships.

Conclusion

For many decades, global attention has focused on the need to deliver effective health care to all, with special attention to impoverished and disenfranchised communities. This effort is part of a larger concern with widespread social and political inequities. Despite calls for institutions to become more democratic, many communities lack the basic resources to engage in self-determination and to flourish.

In this context, health has become synonymous with overall well-being. Researchers, practitioners, and planners have struggled to find ways to work collaboratively with communities to address the unique personal, social, and physical needs that must be fulfilled to create well-being. However, the very research and intervention protocols, often developed to ensure effective data collection and service delivery, serve as obstacles to authentic community participation. Established practices basically cast communities, particularly those with low resources, as incapable of providing valid knowledge, insight, or action.

Participatory community-based research and intervention methods, although designed to allow local control, must be employed with care. The community cannot simply be understood as the new base of operations for employing the usual assumptions about valid knowledge and facts. Instead, the stories of a community must be considered a valid framework for conducting any research or intervention efforts. Dialogue and interpretation, then, are crucial components for any community-based endeavor. Researchers and practitioners must assume that all communities are capable of engaging in sophisticated analysis of their problems and potential solutions.

Mapping is an ideal process for initiating research or intervention from a participatory community-based perspective. Community maps, however, cannot be created from objective geographic references. On the contrary, maps must be formed to reflect the lived experiences of a community. This goal can be accomplished only with authentic, sustained dialogue among local residents and researchers and practitioners. As the mapping process develops, residents can learn the communication, organizational, and advocacy skills important for self-determination. But the goal of authentic local participation can be realized if research and intervention are focused on understanding communities on their own terms and on establishing democratic relationships that will encourage ongoing dialogue.

References

Awofeso, N. (2004). What's new about the "new public health"? *American Journal of Public Health, 94*(5), 705–709.

Barton, H., & Grant, M. (2011). A review of progress of the European Healthy Cities Programme. *Journal of Urban Health: Bulletin of the New York Academy of Medicine, 90*(S1), s129–s141. doi:10.1007/s11524-011-9649-3.

Berger, P. L., & Luckman, T. (1966). *The social construction of reality: A treatise in the sociology of knowledge.* New York: Doubleday & Co.

Blumenthal, D. S., Hopkins, Y., III, & Yancy, E. (2013). Community-based participatory research: An introduction. In D. S. Blumenthal, R. J. DiClemente, R. L. Brauthwaite, & S. S. Smith (Eds.), *Community-based participatory health research: Issues, methods, and translation to practice* (2nd ed., pp. 1–34). New York: Springer Publishing.

Brown, P. (1997). Popular epidemiology revisited. *Current Sociology, 45*(3), 137–156.

Campbell, E., Henly, J. R., Elliott, D. S., & Irwin, K. (2009). Subjective constructions of neighborhood boundaries: Lessons from a qualitative study of four neighborhoods. *Journal of Urban Affairs, 31*(4), 461–490.

Chambers, R. (2006). Participatory mapping and geographic information systems: Whose map? Who is empowered and who disempowered? Who gains and who loses? *The Electronic Journal on Information Systems in Developing Countries, 25*(2), 1–11.

Coulton, C. J., Korbin, J., Chan, T., & Su, M. (2001). Mapping residents' perceptions of neighborhood boundaries: A methodological note. *American Journal of Community Psychology, 29*(2), 371–383.

Coulton, C., Chan, T., & Mikelbank, K. (2011). Finding place in community change initiatives: Using GIS to uncover resident perceptions of their neighborhoods. *Journal of Community Practice, 19*, 10–28.

Coulton, C. J., Jennings, M. Z., & Chan, T. (2013). How big is my neighborhood? Individual and contextual effects on perceptions of neighborhood scale. *American Journal of Community Psychology, 51*, 140–150. doi:10.1007/s10464-012-9550-6.

de Leeuw, E. (2011). Do healthy cities work? A logic of method for assessing impact and outcome of healthy cities. *Journal of Urban Health: Bulletin of the New York Academy of Medicine, 89*(2), 271–231. doi:10.1007/s11524-011-9617-y.

de Leeuw, E., Kickbusch, I., Palmer, N., & Spanswick, L. (2015). European healthy cities come to terms with health network governance. *Health Promotion International, 30*(S1), i32–i44. doi:10.1093/heapro/dav040.

Elwood, S. (2006). Negotiating knowledge production: The everyday inclusions, exclusions, and contradictions of participatory GIS research. *The Professional Geographer, 58*(2), 197–208.

Fals Borda, O. (1988). *Knowledge and people's power*. New York: New Horizons Press.

Fals Borda, O. (2013). Action research in the convergence of disciplines. *International Journal of Action Research, 9*(2), 155–167.

Freire, P. (1992). *Pedagogy of the oppressed*. New York: Continuum.

Gray, M., & Ricciardi, W. (2010). From public health to population medicine: The contribution of public health to health care services [Editorial]. *European Journal of Public Health, 20*(4), 366–367. doi:10.1093/eurpub/ckq091.

Greco, G., Lorgelly, P., & Yamabhai, I. (2016). Outcomes in economic evaluations of public health interventions in low- and middle-income countries: Health, capabilities and subjective well-being. *Health Economics, 25*(Suppl. 1), 83–96. doi:10.1002/hec.3302.

Hawthorne, T. L., & Kwan, M. (2011). Using GIS and perceived distance to understand the unequal geographies of healthcare in lower-income urban neighborhoods. *The Geographic Journal, 178*(1), 18–30.

International Fund for Agricultural Development (IFAD). (2009). *Good practices in participatory mapping, a review prepared for IFAD*. Rome: IFAD.

Kickbusch, I. (2003). The contribution of the World Health Organization to the new public health and health promotion. *American Journal of Public Health, 93*(3), 383–388.

Kieffer, C. (1984). Citizen empowerment: A developmental perspective. In J. Rappaport & R. Hess (Eds.), *Studies in empowerment: Steps toward understanding and action* (pp. 9–36). New York: Haworth Press.

Kindig, D. (2007). Understanding population health terminology. *The Milbank Quarterly, 85*(1), 139–161.

Kindig, D., & Stoddart, G. (2003). What is population health? *American Journal of Public Health, 93*(3), 380–383.

Kirschenbaum, J., & Corburn, J. (2012). Community mapping and digital technology. In M. Minkler (Ed.), *Community organizing and community building for health and welfare* (3rd ed., pp. 444–453). New Brunswick: Rutgers University Press.

Krieger, N. (2001). Theories for social epidemiology in the 21st century: An ecosocial approach. *International Journal of Epidemiology, 30*, 668–677.

Krieger, N. (2009). Putting health inequities on the map: Social epidemiology meets medical/health geography—An ecosocial perspective. *GeoJournal, 74*(2), 87–97.

Murphy, J. (2014). *Community-based interventions: Philosophy and action*. New York: Springer.

Murphy, J. W., Franz, B. A., & Callaghan, K. A. (2015). Is community-based work compatible with data collection? *Journal of Sociology and Social Welfare, XLII*(4), 9–21.

Photis, Y. N. (2016). Disease and health care disparities: Mapping trends and patterns in GIS. *Health Science Journal, 10*(3), 1–8.

Sampson, R. J., Morenoff, J. D., & Gannon-Rowley, T. (2002). Assessing "neighborhood effects": Social processes and new directions in research. *Annual Review of Sociology, 28*, 443–478.

Schutz, A. (1967). *The phenomenology of the social world*. Chicago: Northwestern University Press.

Solomon, B. B. (1976). *Black empowerment: Social work in oppressed communities*. New York: Columbia University Press.

Stokes, B., Villanueva, G., Bar, F., & Ball-Rokeach, S. (2015). Mobile design as neighborhood acupuncture: Activating the storytelling networks of South Los Angeles. *Journal of Urban Technology, 22*(3), 55–77.

Weick, K. E. (1976). Educational institutions as loosely coupled systems. *Administrative Science Quarterly, 21*, 1–19.

World Health Organization. (1978, September 6–12). *Declaration of Alma-Ata*. International Conference on Primary Health Care, Alma-Ata, USSR.

World Health Organization. (1986). *Ottawa Charter for health promotion*. Geneva: World Health Organization.

Chapter 8
Training Physicians with Communities

David Laubli, Daniel Skinner, and Kyle Rosenberger

Introduction and Background: Why Community-Based Medicine?

The last decade has seen a groundswell of scholarly support for rooting health care in communities (Farmer et al. 2006; Wallerstein and Duran 2006; Israel et al. 2010). Despite an emerging consensus that community-based medicine is well positioned to reduce inequalities in access, improve outcomes, and reduce aggregate costs, American health-care institutions have been slow to adapt. Change, however, is occurring. American hospitals, for example, are morphing from isolated medical campuses into centers that are increasingly integrated into communities. Regardless of the partisan perspectives from which they arise, health policy proposals often include at least components of community-based health care.

Medical schools are also beginning to change. Many schools are redefining optimal training spaces to include not only hospitals but private practices, community

---

The authors would like to acknowledge support for this research provided by Ohio University's Research and Scholarly Advancement Fellowship. The authors also thank Dr. Berkeley Franz for helpful research assistance.

D. Laubli (✉)
Ohio University Heritage College of Osteopathic Medicine, Athens, OH, USA
e-mail: dl583914@ohio.edu

D. Skinner
Department of Social Medicine, Ohio University Heritage College of Osteopathic Medicine, Athens, OH, USA
e-mail: skinnerd@ohio.edu

K. Rosenberger
Ohio University Office of Instructional Innovation and Heritage College of Osteopathic Medicine, Ohio University, Athens, OH, USA
e-mail: rosenbek@ohio.edu

health centers and clinics, and even neighborhood schools (Chen et al. 2012). A cursory analysis indicates that many US medical schools acknowledge not only the importance of training students in community settings but also the benefit of preparing students to work collaboratively with patients in communities. This latter approach, which emphasizes the participation of communities in health care, is known as community-based medical education (CBME). While many schools have long encouraged students to engage in one-off or elective experiences in these spaces, the major change with which this chapter is concerned is the extent to which CBME is being carried out earlier and with greater intentionality and institutional support, especially as a formal or required curricular goal.

But how prevalent are these programs and how many schools are *actively* undertaking them? This chapter seeks to accomplish three goals. First, we describe CBME's conceptual foundations and contrast them with historical tendencies to isolate medical education from communities. Second, we present findings from our analysis of CBME in American medical schools that offer a broad snapshot of CBME programs. Third, we explain what would be required were increased investments in CBME made in a widespread and meaningful way. This shift in education is important for the development of effective approaches to medicine that are responsive to community needs, while also addressing workforce shortages in primary and community health care.

Theoretical Foundations of Community-Based Medical Education

CBME aims to immerse medical students in collaborative community settings, in addition to hospital or traditional learning spaces (Hamad 1991). Approaching at least the third decade in which scholars have touted the potential of this model to transform how clinicians are trained, CBME is a fast-developing paradigm with a continuously growing evidence base and many institutions that are investing and reorganizing their fundamental philosophies to accommodate CBME's promise.

A key moment in this history was the release of an influential World Health Organization (WHO) report in 1987, entitled "Community-based Education of Health Personnel." This report detailed an imperative to train future clinicians – especially in primary care – both in and with communities. Especially noteworthy is that CBME programs should have learning activities related to planned educational goals and objectives and be introduced early in the students' medical education. The report also stressed the importance of CBME programs being continuous across the entirety of students' education, mainstreamed into the formal curriculum, and to not be relegated to electives or what scholars often call the "hidden curriculum" (Billings et al. 2011). Additionally, work performed in these community clinical spaces must be substantive and distinguished from traditional fieldwork by being immersive and affording students ample time to understand the social and cultural lifeworlds of the local communities. WHO also emphasizes the mutuality of these educational experiences, thereby insisting they benefit and meaningfully involve both the community and students (See Table 8.1).

Table 8.1 World Health Organization principles for community-based education programs

Principle 1: The students' activities should relate to planned educational goals and objectives; both the students and the teachers must have a clear understanding of the purpose of the activities and the expected results
Principle 2: The activities should be introduced very early in the educational experience
Principle 3: They must continue throughout the educational program
Principle 4: They must be viewed not as peripheral or casual experiences but as a standard, integral, and continuing part of the educational process
Principle 5: The students' work during training must be "real work" that is related to their educational needs and also forming part of the requirements for obtaining a degree
Principle 6: There is a marked difference between the objectives of a community-based education program and those of traditional fieldwork. The students are fully exposed to the social and cultural environment and thus come to understand the important elements of community life and the relationship of those elements to health-related factors and activities. The program must be of clear benefit to both the student and the community. This implies that the community must be actively involved in the educational program

These principles are reinforced by more recent medical education literature. Howe (2002), for example, emphasizes the importance of planned curricular goals and objectives for CBME programs while also indicating the need for students to become fully immersed in the communities in which they are learning. Immersion within communities, as indicated by Worley (2002), helps broaden students' perspectives while enabling them to develop relationships with community members. Kelly et al. (2014) extend this principle of relationship development in CBME by describing the benefits of the student-preceptor partnership. "Students in CBME placements," they note, "witness and are influenced by leadership roles rural doctors and other health professionals have within their community. They learn about primary care from a broad societal perspective as their preceptors participate in public health programs, health promotion campaigns, and advocate to change the social determinants of health within their communities." Such participation also reinforces the tenet of CBME that programs be mutually beneficial for both students and community (WHO 1987).

To critically understand CBME, this idea should be differentiated from related concepts such as "community-oriented education." Magzoub and Schmidt (2000) define CBME as "…a means of achieving educational relevance to community needs and, consequently, serves as a way of implementing a community-oriented education program." Hamad (1991) argues that CBME aims to train "community-orientated doctors who are willing and able to serve their communities and deal effectively with health problems at the primary, secondary and tertiary level," but adds that "The aim is not to produce community medicine specialists or a new category of health specialists, but to respond to the needs of the community concerned." Similarly, Ladhani et al. (2013) describe CBME as a community-focused instructional approach, "…in which not only students, but also faculty members, are actively involved throughout the educational experience." Accordingly, Geiger (2002), perhaps the most influential theorist of community-based paradigms, detailed the achievements of a community health center that trained health professions students alongside community members with the aim of assessing local health problems.

Since the advent of the famous Flexner Report of 1910, American medical education has been structured mostly with 2 years of didactic and skills training and two subsequent years of "rotations" in clinical spaces (Starr 1982; Cooke et al. 2006). During this period, students generally learned "…the complete hospital admission history and physical examination and managing ward rotations." This training was premised on the idea "that learning the complete hospital admission history and physically examining and managing ward patients with their rapidly exchanging, complex illnesses was the basic first step in quality clinical training" (Margolis 2000). Yet, during the latter part of the era, a number of medical schools contemplated the advantages of training and educating medical students in community-based settings, as opposed to exclusively in hospital-based locations.

Despite progress, however, the move toward CBME remains incomplete. A systematic review of CBME conducted by Hunt et al. (2011) found that the fast-growing body of scholarly articles tends to focus on five key themes. Specifically, they found enthusiasm for CBME by educators, evidence of significant heterogeneity in projects, and an emphasis on community experiences as valued equally to traditional medical education. Less optimistically, however, they found a lack of inclusion of community members in identifying local health priorities and a lack of emphasis on reciprocity in the transfer of knowledge between students and the community.

Recent medical education literature emphasizes increasingly the importance of earlier and more contact with patients, including in students' first year (Worley et al. 2004; Van Schalkwyk et al. 2014; Strasser 2015), with particular benefits in the cultivation of empathy (Pedersen 2010; Wenrich et al. 2013), cultural competency skills (Kripalani et al. 2006), and appreciation for team-based care (Howe 2001; Ladhani et al. 2013). Many scholarly works published on CBME detail the nature and scope of fledgling CBME programs around the world, bringing a theoretical shape to such programs. Taken as a whole, this scholarly foundation constitutes a sustained defense of the value of CBME and provides a range of theoretical approaches for establishing and assessing these programs (Sturmberg et al. 2001; Kennedy 2006; Dehaven et al. 2011; Latessa et al. 2015; Stricklin 2016).

While the majority of scholarship documents the benefits of training clinicians in community settings, this change does not mean there are no significant challenges. Doucet and colleagues' study (2014) of the Dalhousie Health Mentors Program, which emphasizes collaborative approaches for the care of patients with chronic conditions, found that the program faced hurdles in the areas of curriculum integration, team composition, and effectiveness of learning assignments. Morrison and Watt (2003) also temper their enthusiasm for CBME by noting a range of challenges in implementing and scaling such programs. Studies, such as Farnsworth, Frantz, and McCune's "Community-based distributive medical education: Advantaging society" (2012), identify challenges in workforce development, especially concerning funding, for CBME.

While the existing literature on CBME is vast and growing, this work tends to center either on fleshing out the theoretical framework for CBME or on case studies of particular programs. Although some of these case studies are of American medical schools, the vast preponderance of scholarship remains non-American, with a particularly large representation of Australian schools, where CBME first took hold on a large scale. To provide a macrolevel picture of such programs in the USA, this chapter aims to provide readers with an overview of American CBME programs.

Methods

To map the current landscape of CBME in the USA, an extensive Internet search of medical school web sites was undertaken for this project. In the attempt to better understand commitments to CBME programs at American medical schools, data points were collected at points such as school demographics; religious, public, or other affiliations; racial demographics; and beyond. Based on these categories, focus was directed to whether or not schools mentioned specifically community-based training in their mission statements, are affiliated with a community health clinic, require training with underserved populations, and offer specific programs that would qualify as CBME. These programs were also analyzed with regard to whether they require training "in" versus "with" local communities. Table 8.2 summarizes the types of programs found in American medical schools.

Two hundred five medical school campuses were surveyed, with an average enrollment of 597 students. Of these, 43% are private, 32% are located in medically underserved areas, and 7% are religiously affiliated. Twenty-eight schools require underserved clinical rotations, but only four mention both communities and the underserved specifically in their mission statements (11 mention only communities and eight mention only underserved). This finding may suggest that though institutions may not view these programs as part of their explicit mission, they are sometimes an inherent part of what they do, perhaps due to geographical location.

A complicating factor in analyzing these data is that many institutions have multiple campuses. In this analysis, multiple campuses are considered separate entities since different opportunities are often afforded to students at these

Table 8.2 Types of community health training offered in American medical schools

Community health special programs	Community-based health special programs
Scholarship/research on the health of underserved populations	Community health center training
Mobile clinics	Service learning opportunities
Free clinics	Community-based participatory research or other community-engaged projects
Student-run clinics	Interprofessional community-based partnerships (e.g., training with community health workers)
School clinics/youth outreach	Community-based preceptors
Health fairs	Mini medical school

different locations. Indiana University, however, has eight campuses that provide classroom training, and although they have separate curriculums, none of them appears to offer distinctly different programs with regard to community health. By contrast, the six campuses at the University of Texas Medical School were clearly founded with different purposes in mind, and some of them (Galveston and San Antonio especially) do emphasize CBME, while others do not. Other schools offer programs that cannot specifically be designated as "campuses" but represent significant efforts that are difficult to categorize alongside the other data. Despite these challenges, the findings offer an important overview of the state of CBME in the USA.

Findings

This web-based study evaluated 205 medical school campuses with an average enrollment size of 597. Private schools made up 43% of the schools, and 57% were public. Of the 205, 65 (32%) are located in medically underserved areas. 15 (or 7%) are religiously affiliated.

One hundred sixty-three schools (79%) report having some form of community clinic, often partially or fully run and managed by students. Twenty-eight schools (14%) report requiring students to rotate into underserved areas. Of these 28 schools, it should be added, 10 (37%) are located in medically underserved areas, which means that being located in such areas seems to be related to having curricula that reflect a commitment to CBME. Nineteen of the 28 schools are private (68%), thus indicating that 21% of private schools require training with or in underserved communities, compared to 8% of public schools. Three of the 28 that require underserved rotations are religiously affiliated.

Many schools require training with underserved populations through longitudinal preceptorships with community physicians during students' first or second years. Others accomplish this goal through their primary care or family medicine clinical rotations during the third year. Of those schools that do not require such training for all students, many offer tracks in rural and underserved health, often supported by scholarships. At some schools, clinical rotation sites are located in underserved or rural areas, and students end up training there as a function of assignment rather than intentional CBME. Other schools are located in and surrounded by counties that are classified as underserved, thereby making such training almost a default. But ascertaining the depth of these schools' commitments, or the reach of these programs into their student bodies, is difficult from college web sites.

The analysis of school mission statements also revealed important differences in programs. Of the 205 mission statements evaluated, 73 (35%) mentioned communities, 32 (16%) mentioned underserved populations, and 20 (10%) mentioned both. Of those mentioning both, 55% are located in medically underserved areas.

A Closer Look at Five Programs

Having provided a wide-lens picture of CBME in the USA, valuable insights are derived from examining the approaches being taken by some of the schools analyzed. While highlighting five programs, this analysis is not intended to suggest that other programs do not have well-developed and innovative CBME programs. The following descriptions are offered merely as an example of the kind of programs that are taking place across medical institutions in the USA:

1. *The Edward Via College of Osteopathic Medicine* (VCOM) is a private, non-profit school with a slightly larger-than-average enrollment, and is located in a mental health and primary care shortage area. VCOM's mission statement identifies its aim "to prepare globally-minded, community-focused physicians to meet the needs of rural and medically underserved populations and promote research to improve human health." VCOM's Appalachian outreach program allows students at its three regional campuses – in Blacksburg, Virginia; Spartanburg, South Carolina; and Auburn, Alabama – to gain experience in public and environmental health and provide care for patients living in poor socio-economic conditions. The web site notes, "Medical outreach experiences are a key component in educating students to provide healthcare in challenging environments." VCOM requires engagement with communities, while providing STEM training to local schools as part of a commitment to reaching rural and otherwise disadvantaged students, and a "Mini Med School" where VCOM students and faculty host programs that promote healthy behaviors and prevent at-risk behaviors.
2. *The University of Maryland School of Medicine,* a public school with above-average enrollment (676), is located in a medically underserved and mental health shortage area of Baltimore, with a household median income significantly below state averages (city-data.com). Despite the absence of CBME in its mission statement, the school requires a 4-week rural experience in the fourth year. Impressively, in addition, over a third of University of Maryland students are part of the school's primary care track, a collaborative effort funded by the US Health Resources and Services Administration that enables medical students to learn about caring for the underserved in Maryland and to work directly in areas of the state that have the greatest need for doctors. In the first 2 years, students spend a half-day per month with primary care faculty members in parts of rural Maryland. In their first summer, students work 80 h with a doctor in one of several underserved areas in the state. The school's popular "Mini Med School" comprises five weekly sessions designed to help Baltimore residents improve their health and well-being and raise public awareness about biomedical research. This mini school helps give lay audiences a better understanding of the terms and concepts used in the biomedical sciences and the importance of research.
3. *The West Virginia University School of Medicine*, a public school in Morgantown, West Virginia, has a class size of 428. Interestingly, considering that the school

is located in the poorest state in the nation, the school is not located in a medically underserved area, though many clinical training sites are in those places. Like the University of Maryland, the West Virginia University School of Medicine's short mission statement does not mention the underserved but focuses on West Virginian communities in general. This mission statement emphasizes that the school "improves the lives of the people of West Virginia and beyond through excellence in patient care, education, research, and service to our communities." Substantive commitments include 100 h of required community service and a mandatory 4-week rural health rotation in the fourth year, with sites across rural and underserved parts of West Virginia.

4. *Campbell University School of Osteopathic Medicine (CUSOM)* is a new private, Christian-affiliated, nonprofit school in Lillington, North Carolina. CUSOM was founded to combat significant workforce shortages in the state, especially in primary care, including one county that did not have even one physician (Fraher and Spero 2015). The school has a larger-than-average enrollment of 648 and is located in a medically underserved area. The mission statement of this school identifies its central goals, "to educate and prepare community-based osteopathic physicians in a Christian environment, to care for the rural and underserved populations in North Carolina, the Southeastern United States and the nation." CUSOM requires a full month of rural underserved training, which is supplemented by (and not, as is common, a replacement for) a separate family practice rotation. Evoking evidence that the best predictor of becoming a rural family physician is rural birth (Owen et al. 2007), CUSOM does extensive outreach to rural high schools (Porter-Rockwell 2013).

5. *The University of Washington School of Medicine* (UW), a public school in Seattle with 1025 students, is not located in an underserved area and does not require students to train in underserved areas. UW is significant because of the numerous ways opportunities are provided for students to engage with communities. In recognition of "many students' desire to work with underserved populations," UW has undertaken the arduous work of creating five curricular "pathways" through which students can learn to work with five specific groups: Hispanics, American Indians, non-American or "global" populations, LGBTQ persons, and the underserved. UW's participation in the WWAMI Regional Medical Education Program, a collaboration with four states that lack medical schools (Wyoming, Alaska, Montana, and Idaho), is intended to increase the number of primary care physicians and address workforce shortages in rural areas. Programs available throughout the region include a 4-week Rural/Underserved Opportunities Program held in the summer between a student's first and second year, a 6-month WWAMI Rural Integrated Training Experience, and a four-year Targeted Rural Underserved Track where students train in and with rural communities.

Discussion and Recommendations for Future Investments in CBME

These findings reveal a myriad of American medical education programs that evoke various tenets of CBME. One of the difficulties in undertaking a comprehensive assessment of these programs is distinguishing deep commitment to such programs, in which many or all students at a school are trained, as opposed to thinner offerings that may reduce exposure to CBME for a select group of students or as intermittent or elective opportunities. Despite these differences, this study does make clear that most US medical schools are increasingly compelled to acknowledge the importance of communities to training a twenty-first-century workforce of physicians. This finding is a promising signpost that programs deeply invested in CBME are harbingers of a broader movement currently in progress, even if this change is uneven regionally and in many cases slow.

This study is unable, however, to account for institutional motivations in investing in CBME. As noted, schools located in medically underserved areas do seem to take notice of community needs and recognize the benefits and importance of training their students in and sometimes with communities. Those schools whose missions are tethered to community and – more broadly – public workforce needs also appear to recognize the importance of more serious commitments to CBME. In addition, given the history of the osteopathic profession, which from its nineteenth-century inception was concerned with rural and community-based medicine (Gevitz 2004), osteopathic medical schools are more likely to require community-based training than their allopathic counterparts. "Social accountability-related objectives," after all, are a staple of many osteopathic medical schools, codified in their mission statements (Phillips-Madson and Dharamsi 2016). These findings also confirm conclusions from Mullan et al. (2010), namely, that public medical schools tend to have high levels of social commitment. Yet, these findings depart from Mullan and colleagues in that the location of many private medical schools in medically underserved or rural areas often makes them more engaged with these populations.

Since the value of CBME is being increasingly recognized in American medical education, most schools are well positioned to conceptualize a larger vision for a mobilization around CBME's core values, which in turn provide an outlook for future physicians. Especially as the USA continues to struggle to meet the needs of those with new access to healthcare coverage and addresses the needs of those who still lack these services, the ability to train physicians who are willing (and incentivized) to practice in medically underserved areas and in collaboration with local communities is paramount.

Accordingly, CBME's critical role within the larger picture of American health care should put persistent and increased pressure on American medical schools to think about what role their students will play in the new and emerging health-care landscape. As Howe (2002) helpfully explains, this process will require that medical schools consider a new range of themes, such as the importance of becoming (and remaining) clear on the values that lead to increased involvement in community training, keeping in mind that community-based medical staff (including those in training) are serving simultaneously as role models, attending to trainee culture shock as a pedagogical and practical matter, the importance of assessment, and the fact that students training in these spaces are also agents of social accountability. Howe's recommendations further remind academics and practitioners that engagement in CBME must be intentional, critical, reflective, and culturally aware. Embracing CBME also will require that students be carefully selected for these programs, since future physicians will have to buy into the future of community medicine if they want to train in medical schools that take seriously CBME. For medical schools that offer CBME as a strongly encouraged elective component, this selection may take place from within general student populations. Schools that are committed more deeply to CBME, however, will need to shape their admissions process around the qualities that CBME requires. The latter path would have the potential to more radically shape medical school culture on a national level than the former, thus instituting a major change in how American medical schools select students.

Also emphasized by these findings is the importance of guarding against the more trivial, symbolic, or even public relations angles to which CBME might fall prey. As with all aspects of social engagements that can devolve into photo opportunities, CBME, to be an effective teaching as well as substantive tool for producing certain kinds of physicians, must be cared for and taken seriously. This suggestion means, among other things, that community members must be involved meaningfully and continuously in identifying local health needs and establishing strategic priorities that address these issues and that this process must be a genuine collaboration between medical students and their preceptors and community members and leaders. Perhaps most important, an ethic of reciprocity must stand at the center of such programs.

Conclusion

The study that serves as a foundation of this chapter is intended to be a signpost rather than an exhaustive accounting. Since the data are based primarily on publicly available web site information, they are not able to capture some of the finer details of programs already existing or in progress. Additionally, details are not available that indicate which programs have deep commitments with dedicated staff and appropriate funding to support them and which are more aspirational or partial. Yet, this study can say with certainty that a discursive shift has occurred and continues to be underway, as evidenced by a very large number of medical schools that have gone out of their way to spotlight CBME in their online profiles. This finding is significant considering that web sites are usually the first point of contact with interested students, philanthropists and partners, new hires, and community members. In a strong way, the claim can be made that the web sites analyzed signal a widespread recognition that community medicine must be a central concern of twenty-first-century medical education, yet this change alone is not enough to make CBME the norm or to have a substantive effect on the health of American communities. This change may, in many cases, signal little more than a public projection. But as with all things, the recognition of a problem, or the setting of a course, is a meaningful first step.

References

Billings, M. E., Lazarus, M. W., Curtis, J. R., & Engelberg, R. A. (2011). The effect of the hidden curriculum on resident burnout and cynicism. *Journal of Graduate Medical Education, 3*(4), 503–510.

Chen, C., Chen, F., & Mullan, F. (2012). Teaching health centers: A new paradigm in graduate medical education. *Academic Medicine: Journal of the Association of American Medical Colleges, 87*(12), 1752–1756.

City-Data.com. 21201 zip code (Baltimore, MD) detailed profile. http://www.city-data.com/zips/21201.html

Cooke, M., Irby, D. M., Sullivan, W., & Ludmerer, K. M. (2006). American medical education 100 years after the Flexner report. *New England Journal of Medicine, 355*, 1339–1344.

Dehaven, M. J., Gimpel, N. E., Dallo, F. J., & Billmeier, T. M. (2011). Reaching the underserved through community-based participatory research and service learning: Description and evaluation of a unique medical student training program. *Journal of Public Health Management and Practice, 17*(4), 363–368.

Doucet, S., MacKenzie, D., Loney, E., Godden-Webster, A., Lauckner, H., Brown, P. A., & Packer, T. L. (2014). Curricular factors that unintentionally affect learning in a community-based interprofessional education program: The student perspective. *Journal of Research in Interprofessional Practice & Education, 4*(2), 1–30.

Farmer, P. E., Nizeye, B., Stulac, S., & Keshavjee, S. (2006). Structural violence and clinical medicine. *PLoS Medicine, 3*(10), e449.

Farnsworth, T. J., Frantz, A. C., & McCune, R. W. (2012). Community-based distributive medical education: Advantaging society. *Medical Education Online, 17*. doi:10.3402/meo.v17i0.8432.

Fraher, E. P., & Spero, J. C. (2015). *The state of the physician workforce in North Carolina: Overall physician supply will likely be sufficient but is maldistributed by specialty and geography.* The Cecil G, Sheps Center for Health Services Research (UNC). http://www.shepscenter.unc.edu/wp-content/uploads/2015/08/MedicalEducationBrief-ShepsCenter-August20151.pdf

Geiger, H. J. (2002). Community-oriented primary care: A path to community development. *American Journal of Public Health, 92*(11), 1713–1716.

Gevitz, N. (2004). *The DOs: Osteopathic medicine in America*. Baltimore: Johns Hopkins University Press.

Hamad, B. (1991). Community-oriented medical education: What is it? *Medical Education, 25*(1), 16–22.

Howe, A. (2001). Patient-centered medicine through student-centred teaching: A student perspective on the key impacts of community- based learning in undergraduate medical education. *Medical Education, 35*(7), 666–672.

Howe, A. (2002). Twelve tips for community-based medical education. *Medical Teacher, 24*(1), 9–12.

Hunt, J. B., Bonham, C., & Jones, L. (2011). Understanding the goals of service learning and community-based medical education: A systematic review. *Academic Medicine, 86*(2), 246–251.

Israel, B. A., Coombe, C. M., Cheezum, R. R., Schulz, A. J., McGranaghan, R. J., Lichtenstein, R., & Burris, A. (2010). Community-based participatory research: A capacity-building approach for policy advocacy aimed at eliminating health disparities. *American Journal of Public Health, 100*(11), 2094–2102.

Kelly, L., et al. (2014). Community-based medical education: Is success a result of meaningful personal learning experiences? *Education for Health, 27*(1), 47–50.

Kennedy, E. M. (2006). Beyond vertical integration – Community based medical education. *Australian Family Physician, 35*(11), 901–903.

Kripalani, S., Bussey-Jones, J., Katz, M. G., & Genao, I. (2006). A prescription for cultural competence in medical education. *Journal of General Internal Medicine, 21*(10), 1116–1120.

Ladhani, Z., Stevens, F. J., & Scherpbier, A. J. (2013). Competence, commitment and opportunity: An exploration of faculty views and perceptions on community- based education. *BMC Medical Education, 13*, 167.

Latessa, R., Beaty, N., Royal, K., Colvin, G., Pathman, D. E., & Heck, J. (2015). Academic outcomes of a community-based longitudinal integrated clerkships program. *Medical Teacher, 37*(9), 862–867.

Magzoub, M. A., & Schmidt, H. G. (2000). A taxonomy of community-based medical education. *Academic Medicine, 75*(7), 699–707.

Margolis, C. (2000). Community-based medical education. *Medical Teacher, 22*(5), 482–484.

Morrison, J., & Watt, G. (2003). New century, new challenges for community based medical education. *Medical Education, 37*(1), 2–3.

Mullan, F., Chen, C., Petterson, S., Kolsky, G., & Spagnola, M. (2010). The social mission of medical education: Ranking the schools. *Annals of Internal Medicine, 152*, 804–811.

Owen, J. A., Conaway, M. R., Bailey, B. A., & Hayden, G. F. (2007). Predicting rural practice using different definitions to classify medical school applicants as having a rural upbringing. *Journal of Rural Health, 23*(2), 133–140.

Pedersen, R. (2010). Empathy development in medical education – A critical review. *Medical Teacher, 32*(7), 593–600.

Phillips-Madson, R., & Dharamsi, S. (2016). Osteopathic medical education and social accountability. *The Journal of the American Osteopathic Association, 116*, 202–206.

Porter-Rockwell, B. (2013). New Campbell med school trains rural health doctors. *North Carolina Health News*. http://www.northcarolinahealthnews.org/2013/08/23/new-campbell-med-school-trains-rural-health-doctors/

Starr, P. (1982). *The social transformation of american medicine*. New York: Basic Books.

Strasser, R., Worley, P., Cristobal, F., Marsh, D. C., Berry, S., Strasser, S., & Ellaway, R. (2015). Putting communities in the driver's seat: The realities of community-engaged medical education. *Academic Medicine, 90*(11), 1466–1470.

Stricklin, S. M. (2016). Achieving clinical competencies through community-based clinical experiences. *Journal of the American Psychiatric Nurses Association, 22*(4), 291–301.

Sturmberg, J., Reid, A., & Khadra, M. (2001). Community based medical education in a rural area: A new direction in undergraduate training. *Australian Journal of Rural Health, 9*, 14–18.

Van Schalkwyk, S., Bezuidenhout, J., Conradie, H., Fish, T., Kok, N., Van Heerden, B., & De Villiers, M. (2014). 'Going rural': Driving change through a rural medical education innovation. *Rural and Remote Health, 14*(2), 2493.

Wallerstein, N. B., & Duran, B. (2006). Using community-based participatory research to address health disparities. *Health Promotion Practice, 7*, 312–323.

Wenrich, M. D., Jackson, M. B., Wolfhagen, I., Ramsey, P. G., & Scherpbier, A. J. J. (2013). What are the benefits of early patient contact? – A comparison of three preclinical patient contact settings. *BMC Medical Education, 13*, 80.

World Health Organization. (1987). http://apps.who.int/iris/bitstream/10665/41714/1/WHO_TRS_746.pdf

Worley, P. O. (2002). Relationships: A new way to analyse community based medical education? (part one). *Education for Health: Change in Learning & Practice, 15*(2), 117–128.

Worley, P., Prideaux, D., Strasser, R., March, R., & Worley, E. (2004). What do medical students actually do on clinical rotations? *Medical Teacher, 26*(7), 594–598.

Chapter 9
A Community-Based Approach to Primary Health Care

Khary K. Rigg, Doug Engelman, and Jesús Ramirez

Defining Primary Health Care

Primary health care (PHC) is a term that describes an approach to health policy and service provision that includes services delivered to individuals, as well as population-level public health functions (Muldoon et al. 2006). According to the United Nations Children's Fund (UNICEF)/World Health Organization's (WHO) Alma-Ata declaration, PHC is essential health care made universally accessible to individuals and families in the community, by means acceptable to them, and at a cost that the community and country can afford (UNICEF and World Health Organization 1978). Moreover, PHC becomes an integral part both of the country's health-care system, indeed, the nucleus, and the overall social and economic development of the community. PHC addresses ideally the most fundamental health concerns of a community, while providing promotive, preventive, curative, supportive, and rehabilitative services according to need. According to the WHO, when properly implemented, PHC constitutes the starting point of a continuing health-care process. In fact, PHC implementation calls for a commitment to the achievement of maximum community and individual self-reliance for health development, which

K.K. Rigg (✉)
Department of Mental Health Law & Policy, University of South Florida, Tampa, FL, USA
e-mail: rigg@usf.edu

D. Engelman
Department of Sociology, University of South Florida, Tampa, FL, USA
e-mail: dengelman@mail.usf.edu

J. Ramirez
Department of Philosophy, University of South Florida, Tampa, FL, USA
e-mail: jesusramirez@mail.usf.edu

includes technical knowledge, training, guidance and supervision, logistic support, supplies, financing, and referral facilities, including institutions where unsolved problems and individual patients can be referred (UNICEF and World Health Organization 1978).

PHC is often conflated with other related concepts, particularly primary care (PC). PC describes a far narrower concept of "family doctor-type" services delivered to individuals (Starfield 1994). PC is the provision of *integrated, accessible health-care services* by *clinicians* who are *accountable* for addressing a large *majority of personal health-care needs*, developing a *sustained partnership* with *patients*, and practicing in the *context of family and community*. This concept stresses the importance of the patient-clinician relationship in the context of the patient's family and community and as facilitated and augmented by teams and integrated delivery systems (Institute of Medicine [IOM] 1996). Nonetheless, in PC, health care is controlled by physicians, with communities only periodically consulted.

Primary Health Care: A Challenge to Tradition

PHC is quite a departure from the traditional approach to health-care delivery. In fact, there was initially significant resistance to PHC since this approach represented a true paradigm shift in thinking about health (Van Lerberghe 2008). Clearly, the proper application of a PHC model has profound consequences, not only throughout the health sector but also for other social and economic domains at both the national and the community levels. However, with change usually comes resistance. Attempts to ensure a more equitable distribution of health resources have met with resistance from both political and professional groups (Cueto 2004). Furthermore, the introduction of new technology may arouse opposition from traditional medical practitioners and the medical industry. Obstacles such as these can be overcome, if anticipated in advance. The most important factors in promoting PHC, and overcoming such obstacles, are a strong political will, and support at local and national levels, reinforced by a firm national strategy (UNICEF and World Health Organization 1978).

Specific "antidotes" may be employed in this battle. For example, often reticent health professionals can be recruited by involving them in the development phase. In doing so, they can be assured that they are not *relinquishing* medical functions but instead are *gaining* health responsibilities (Gofin and Gofin 2005). In the same way, resistance by the general public can be diffused by discussions in the communities and the media. These discussions should make people understand that PHC is realistic, and desirable, since this strategy provides affordable health care for everyone, in a spirit of social justice, as opposed to models that promote social inequality by remaining physically and financially unattainable in the poorest communities (UNICEF & World Health Organization 1978).

Alma-Ata: The Origins of Primary Health Care

Some argue that through the experience of providing for the medical needs of both combatants and local populations during WWII, health-care delivery changed (Rifkin et al. 1988). Others cite the experiences of missionaries and the development of "rural medical services" that led to a greater need for localized medical care delivery systems (Peterson 1998). All of these factors, and more, have influenced a change from the Western model of "hospital-based" health care, with an emphasis on treatment, to a model that emphasizes prevention.

The concept of PMC emerged in the final decades of the Cold War. The so-called vertical model that had widely been used in malaria eradication by US agencies, and the WHO since the late 1950s, began to come under criticism (Unger 1986). Important contributors to the debate over global health and development, such as John Bryant, questioned the transplantation of the hospital-based health-care system to developing countries, particularly the lack of emphasis on prevention (Bryant 1969). Bryant, clearly recognizing the vast inequalities in health-care delivery in the world's less economically developed countries, argues that a significant number of the world's population, perhaps more than half, have no access to health care. Moreover, for many of the rest, the care they receive is poorly targeted or inadequate.

Carl Taylor, founder and chairman of the Department of International Health at Johns Hopkins University, suggested that Indian rural medicine could be a general model for poor countries (Taylor 1976). Similarly, Kenneth W. Newell argued that a strict health sectorial approach is ineffective (Newell 1975). In addition, the 1974 Canadian Lalonde Report proposed *four* determinants of health. In addition to health services, the report identified biology, the environment, and lifestyle as being equally important in assessing the health status of poor countries (Cueto 2004).

Numerous studies from outside the global medical community were also influential in challenging the assumption that health resulted from the transference of technology, or more doctors and services (Cueto 2004). British historian Thomas McKeown argued that the overall health of the population is less related to medical advances than to standards of living and nutrition (McKeown 1976). More aggressively, Ivan Illich agreed in *Medical Nemesis* that medicine is not only irrelevant, perhaps even detrimental, because medical doctors expropriated health from the public (Cueto 2004).

Aside from the numerous experts who call for fundamental changes in global health-care initiatives, other "real-world" experiences were having an impact. For example, the Christian Medical Commission (CMC), created in the 1960s by medical missionaries, began to emphasize the training of local workers and equipping them with essential drugs and simple medical techniques (Peterson 1998). In fact, the CMC is often credited with coining the term primary health care.

Another important inspiration for primary health care was the global popularity of the massive expansion of rural medical services in communist China, especially the "barefoot doctors" (Tollman 1991). They were a diverse array of village health workers who lived in the communities they served, stressed rural rather than urban health care and preventive rather than curative services, and combined Western and traditional medicines.

In response to this changing medical care landscape, the WHO and UNICEF held the landmark event, an International Conference on Primary Health Care that took place at Alma-Ata, Kazakhstan, in September of 1978 (Cueto 2004). This conference is regarded widely as the birthplace of the PHC model. Over 3000 delegates from 134 countries, and 67 international organizations attended the conference, and 150 countries accepted the final declaration (Rifkin and Walt 1986).

Two of the principle objectives, established at the opening of the conference, in the form of a challenge offered to those in attendance by WHO Director General, Halfdan Mahler, were (1) the willingness to introduce radical changes into existing health-care delivery systems, and properly support PHC as the overriding health priority, and (2) a willingness to fight the political and technical battles required to overcome any social and economic obstacles and professional resistance to the universal introduction of PHC.

The conference's *Declaration of Alma-Ata* was overwhelmingly approved. Three key ideas are found within the declaration:

1. The use of *appropriate* technology – too often technology employed in poor or remote areas was overly sophisticated or expensive or even irrelevant to the needs of the population. Additionally, the Western-oriented model of "urban hospitals" was perceived as promoting a "dependent mentality," was too expensive, and often served a minority of the population.
2. Opposition to medical elitism – this idea resulted from the disapproval of the overspecialization of health personnel in developing countries and of "top-down" health campaigns. Instead, training of lay health personnel and community participation was stressed. The need to work with local traditions and practitioners such as shamans and midwives was emphasized.
3. The concept of health as a tool for socioeconomic development – health care was not considered to be an isolated element and short term but should be viewed as a part of the process of improving overall living conditions and lifestyles.

This idea requires a new way for both public and private institutions to view health-related issues, such as health education, housing, safe water, and basic sanitation. Furthermore, the connection between health and development has political implications that need to be understood and incorporated into planning. As Mahler proclaimed, "we could become the avant-garde of an international conscience for social development" (Mahler 1975).

Combining the Primary Health-Care Model into a Community-Based Philosophy

PHC is essential health care made accessible to individuals and families in their communities and is an integral part of a community's social *and* economic well-being. PHC is the initial, and therefore most important, point of contact for most individuals in the community and thus constitutes the first element of an ongoing health-care process. Moreover, PHC is designed to be affordable, focused on the specific needs of the community, high quality, decentralized (thus adaptable to local conditions), and staffed by appropriately trained local professionals (Muldoon et al. 2006).

Some scholars, however, are rethinking the ways that health-care delivery is conceptualized at the community level. For example, Anderson et al. (2003) argue that social factors, such as resources, accessibility, and seriousness of a problem, which are valued and prioritized contribute greatly to whether treatment will be sought by individuals. Rather than trying to rationalize their decisions on purely epidemiological factors, individuals base their actions on expectations that relate to collective memories, past experiences, and the perceived chances of success (Rigg et al. 2014).

Direct involvement in a community, accordingly, helps to insure that epidemiological assessments are informed by the concepts and judgments used by individuals to arrange their everyday affairs, including their health status. The general point of community-based epidemiology is that health status has little meaning divorced from the biography of a community (Murphy 2015). Viewed from this perspective, adopting a PHC model, with an emphasis on biology, the environment, and socioeconomic factors becomes effective in addressing the issues of access and efficacy at the community level.

However, before PHC can become truly community based, an important question is why the community has been elevated in importance, including the theoretical justification for this elevation. The origins of the biomedical model began in the early seventeenth century (Hewa and Hetherington 1995). Originally, the biomedical model (also known as the medical model) was a biologically reductionist perspective of the body (Engel 1977). Anything that ailed an individual could be reduced to some sort of physiological malady. As a result, hardly any attention was paid to the surrounding environment and how persons are psychologically and socially integrated, active, and responsive to their environment.

Ontologically, where ontology is the analysis of being, the medical model identified two kinds: mind and body. This model proposed a dualism. This dualism was and continues to be influential, and goes back to René Descartes' seventeenth century claim, "I think, therefore, I am" (Descartes 1637/1999, p. 25). For philosophers like Descartes, the relationship between the mind and the body was like that of a ghost in a machine. In the end, the mind controls the body. Medical experts then divided their analysis. One group of experts interrogated the mind, while other experts analyzed the body. This ontological dualism of mind and body present in the biomedical model continues today where you see the mind and body isolated from each other in the attempt to identify the causes of maladies.

This individualistic view, which divides the person, sets up a paradigm that is reductionistic. For example, the patient is not embodied and enmeshed in an environment. Rather, the patient becomes an object to be fixed by the expert practitioner. "Thus the biomedical model embraces both reductionism, the philosophical view that complex phenomena are ultimately derived from single primary principles, and mind-body dualism, the doctrine that separates the mental from the somatic" (Engel 1977, p. 130). To counter these shortcomings, a community-based approach to PHC has the capacity to work more effectively to the extent that this method can be extracted from the philosophical underpinnings of the biomedical model. That is, in the framework provided by a theoretical foundation, PHC might be able to finally come to fruition.

In the biomedical model, doctor and patient are involved in a hierarchical relationship whereby one person has the expertise and the other reports an injury. The doctor then summons his or her knowledge to "fix" the patient. In a schema such as this, the perspective of patients is often obscured. With a replacement theoretical foundation, such as phenomenology, perhaps medicine can become more attuned to desires of communities. Furthermore, without a final removal of the influence of the medical model, the real impact of PHC may be tempered.

Phenomenology and Primary Health Care

Maurice Merleau-Ponty is one of the most well-known phenomenologists who focused on the body and popularized the notion of embodiment (Audi 2006). His work can help shed some light on the theoretical trappings of medicine that practitioners encounter with the mind-body ontological binary. The motivation behind phenomenology is that people, through a rigorous descriptive analysis of their experiences, can push aside any attitudes that would usurp their understanding of the phenomenon in question. At work here is an assumption that there is a meaning to phenomena that should not be distorted. The goals for phenomenologists, therefore, are to simply understand the world, to become more intimate with one's environment, and to resist the use of unquestioned attitudes that bias experience.

In the case of a medical scenario, these goals already prove to be potentially helpful for reevaluating the flaws and attributes of PHC. Already present in this phenomenological method is a critique of the biomedical model that primes people to understand patients as single objects that consist of a mind and body, isolated from the environment and other people. This concretization of a human being, while sometimes scientifically fruitful, limits the scope of analysis with regard to helping patients and communities in need. Thus, even if the community-based PHC model is markedly different from the biomedical one, and they still share the same philosophical foundation, appropriate medical solutions may still not be recognized. Therefore, a phenomenological approach, in the vein of Merleau-Ponty's *Phenomenology of Perception*, might be helpful as a new philosophical basis for PHC (Merleau-Ponty 2012). In this work, he wanted to introduce a version of experience that included the way bodies assist to set the conditions for experience. As a result, relationships, environments, modes of communication, and bodily experiences are a part of understanding every phenomenon, even health.

Experiences matter, but their meaning is both ambiguous and dynamic. As Alcoff (2006, p. 11) stresses, "We are embodied, yet not reduced to physical determinates imagined as existing outside of our place in culture and history." Alcoff's assessment of Merleau-Ponty suggests the value of a testimonial approach that relies on a patient's analysis of their situational experience. Additionally, there is an important inference to be made here: if a patient's testimony is important to understanding the best ways to provide care, then those close to this person, be they family or close members of the community, are equally important in this process. Once the experiences become the focus, no longer should practitioners be concerned with representations of the body but with the situational context and experiences of the patient. This point is crucial to this particular method. With this emphasis now on embodiment, PHC may be able to overcome obstacles that were present to providing proper health care.

One example of a community-based approach that carefully attends to the body in the environment is in Richard Tangwa's work on African Bioethics (Tangwa 2010). He proposes an idea called "moral pluralism." Moral pluralism evaluates individual needs through dialogical community engagement with a person's families that is consistent with the goals of PHC. Here, a phenomenological approach that is already instantiated in African communitarian values becomes a basis for health care that focuses on community. He notes that the main difference between the care allotted to patients in African and Western countries such as the United States is that preventive and curative needs are primary, while in the United States treatment is too often linked to cost-benefit assessments. A patient in Africa, accordingly, will more likely have a treatment plan that emphasizes lifestyle changes related, for example, to eating, sleeping, and exercising.

Especially important is that these non-technological changes are not the outcome of a romanticized notion of Africa that many people adopt. While metropolitan parts of Africa do wrestle with access to technology, non-technological solutions are more of a product of community-based thinking that promotes a practical engagement with others to help solve health issues in a more expedient and effective manner. The problem, Tangwa believes, is that Western care is tied to markets rather than communities. Nonetheless, despite the differences that he points out, a community-based philosophy of care has proven to be effective in not only Africa but in the United States (Tangwa 2010). The movement toward community-based care was brought about in Africa to center the care goals around a patient's experiences, which required communication with the patient's families, social workers, schools, counselors, nurses, doctors, and other relevant practitioners. This change was important because the previous practice of PHC was influenced by the medical model, and thus a slew of patients was supposed to be treated as entities to be repaired and managed.

A community-based perspective on PHC might incorporate elements drawn from phenomenology, moral pluralism, and ethics of care. This strategy has an intersectional quality that centers on a holistic conception of the human that connects persons to their communities. Each of these positions provides a similar sketch of the human as part of a network of relations. If the phenomenological approach is followed, and the theoretical vestiges of the biomedical model avoided, PHC can escape from the individualistic trappings that have hampered this novel approach to medicine. Instead of simply attending to a patient-doctor dichotomy, where health care is focused on a mind-body binary, practitioners can include historical accounts of patients, their personal experiences of illness, and their engagement with communities.

The community-based philosophical approach to PHC involves people not simply as patients to be worked on but subjects who should be actively engaged. The shift opens a possibility for phenomenological testimonials to be integrated into PHC patient-centered solutions. One way of re-conceptualizing primary care from the community standpoint is to draw on various scholars and ideas that speak to the notion of a community (Murphy and Rigg 2014). Literature in disability studies, global bioethics, and marginalized epistemologies already exists that emphasizes the moral rationale for medical practitioners to be culturally competent (Stonington and Ratanakul 2014). Sociological analyses are already engaging the medical field to assess the need for increasing stronger networks in underrepresented communities to create more access to a healthy living (Das et al. 2008). Studies have addressed the need to engage, for example, in order to establish the trust that is necessary for patients and doctors to communicate. In the end, conceptualizing PHC from a phenomenological or morally pluralistic approach can yield great benefits. Reevaluating PHC in this way, rather than through the philosophical foundations of a biomedical version of PHC, can help medical practitioners create more solutions for communities and patients in need.

Moving Primary Health Care Forward

Philosophy clearly plays a big role in determining whether the full potential of PHC will ever be realized. To help achieve this end, three recommendations are made that should move PHC in a more community-based direction. First, narratives (Agnew 2006; Charmaz 1999) are a useful but underutilized approach that reflects the idea that a patient's reality is situational. Illness narratives (Williams 1984), in particular, provide an innovative and effective way of approaching the personal aspects of the illness experience (Ezzy 2000). The norms of a patient's local context, which narratives can help identify, should ideally be used to guide the delivery of care. A course of treatment, in other words, should be driven by the various narratives and storylines in a patient's life and not simply by the results of medical tests or financial constraints (Frank 1998; Rigg and Murphy 2013). For example, narrative approaches are sensitive to the situations of people and can bring into view relevant details of patients' lives that in most cases are of critical importance to treatment success and improved health (Charon 2001; Kleinman and Kleinman 1996).

Narrative medicine, for example, has been receiving some attention as a new model for clinical practice (Charon 2001). This approach to medicine recognizes the value of patients' narratives in practice, research, and education. Proponents of narrative medicine have argued that most medical schools train physicians to treat health problems as simply medical issues, without taking into account the specific psychological and social history of the patient (Remen 2002). Narrative medicine places patients' stories at the center of medical practice and education to encourage a more patient-centered approach to care. Not so much a new specialty as a new frame for clinical care and research, narrative medicine can validate the experience of patients and encourage physician self-reflection, thereby leading to improved health outcomes (Greenhalgh and Hurwitz 1999).

Second, use of visual methods, such as photovoice, can help to make PHC more community grounded (Lopez et al. 2005). Photovoice, in particular, is a method well suited to capturing and conveying the point of view of patients and research participants. Succinctly defined as a process whereby people can identify, represent, and enhance their community through a specific photographic technique, photovoice entails providing individuals with cameras and thus allows them to record, discuss, and communicate to others their realities as seen through their own eyes (Wang et al. 2000; Wang and Burris 1997). The production of a photograph and the photographer's description of the photo provide the foundation for building a shared understanding that can be used as data for research or making health-care decisions (Newman 2010). Photovoice is consistent with the core tenets of community-based research (e.g., empowerment, participation) and PHC.

Photovoice has recently received a great deal of attention from both providers and researchers alike, due to the ability of patients to generate new understanding about health-care experiences and decision-making (Wang et al. 1998). In this way, the identification and documentation of problems (i.e., poor quality of care, barriers to health-care utilization) are made by the participants themselves. Particularly important is that the use of photovoice also provides an opportunity for disenfranchised populations (i.e., homeless, disabled) to share their experiences with the research community, service providers, and policymakers – groups to which these populations typically have little access (Lopez et al. 2005; Rigg et al. 2014). In a recent project, photovoice was used successfully to engage military veterans in communicating their experiences regarding challenges to getting their health-care needs met (True et al. 2014). The data generated by this project not only informed new policy decisions by the Veterans Health Administration but were also used to create a photo exhibit that sensitized providers to how community reintegration experiences impact the health(care) of returning soldiers.

And third, how physicians are trained should be rethought. The clinical education of medical students needs to move further away from academic medical centers and deeper into communities so that physicians are more attuned to the local contexts of their patients (Hensel et al. 1996). Historically, medical students have been trained in settings (e.g., university campuses) that are far removed from the communities of those most in need (Bynum and Porter 2013). To address this issue, there has been a recent push for medical education to become more community sensitive (Strasser et al. 2015). However, medical schools have tried to correct this problem by simply moving training to a new venue. The thinking is that by training more students in community hospitals and clinics, service delivery would automatically become more community based and culturally grounded. But besides a simple change in location, a new orientation to medical education was never adopted, and the overemphasis on technical training still remained.

Medical education today continues to focus heavily on the biomedical aspects of health care, thus resulting in many graduates who are deficient in skills important to clinical practice, including cultural competence. Although cultural competence has become a staple of contemporary medical education (Paul et al. 2014), this concept is often employed in a reductionist manner. Many medical schools seemingly take the position that exposing physicians to static, prepackaged ideas of "culture" will assist them in estimating patient behaviors or preferences in the clinic, thereby diminishing health-care disparities. But the idea that doctors can diagnose patients by spending only a few minutes with them, and then quietly infer their cultural belief system, is reductive and inadequate (Tsai 2016).

Therefore, rather than cultural competence that narrowly views patient preferences as a series of generalized stereotypes, medical schools should embrace frameworks that do not attempt to "fit" patients into preconceived cultural rubrics (Chang et al. 2012). Cultural humility is one such framework (Miller 2009). This approach shifts the focus from doctors to patients and from providers to community members. In other words, cultural humility recognizes the complexity of cultural identity and belief, inaugurates a lifelong commitment to self-evaluation and critique to redress the power imbalances in the physician-patient dynamic, and develops mutually beneficial and non-paternalistic partnerships with communities (Tervalon and Murray-Garcia 1998).

Similarly, structural competency addresses cultural competency's failure to look beyond the doctor-patient dyad to counter inequity (Tsai 2016). Specifically, structural competency contends that many health-related factors previously attributed to culture also represent the downstream consequences of decisions about larger structural contexts, including health-care and food delivery systems, zoning laws, local politics, urban and rural infrastructures, structural racism, or even the very definitions of illness and health (Metzl and Hanson 2014). Both cultural humility and structural competency are important frameworks for preparing student physicians to become competent providers. In view of the need for community-based interventions, these approaches should be adopted by more medical schools as a component of a more overarching reorganization of physician training.

Conclusion

PHC is supposed to include the broadest scope of health care in order to reach patients of all ages, socioeconomic backgrounds, geographic origins, and health conditions. The conceptualization and implementation of PHC, however, have yet to be fully realized. Reevaluating PHC through new theoretical lenses, such as phenomenology or moral pluralism, rather than through the philosophical foundations of biomedicine, can help PHC reach its true potential and work more effectively for everyone. In this way, the initial steps to a more community-oriented PHC are theoretical.

For PHC to become truly community oriented, interventions must move beyond focusing primarily on increasing access to care. At the heart of community-based PHC is a reconceptualization of health-care delivery and planning. Community-based health care does not simply expand access to health services but rather deploys communities to give direction to any health initiatives. Ignoring this realm of agency reduces health care to issues of delivery efficacy. A PHC approach is community based when health plans are designed from the ground up and reflect the everyday lives of community members. Their participation establishes the reality that informs the identification of needs, the development of health interventions, and the criteria for determining a successful program of health services.

References

Agnew, R. (2006). Storylines as a neglected cause of crime. *Journal of Research in Crime and Delinquency, 43*(2), 119–131.
Alcoff, L. M. (2006). *Visible identities: Race, gender, and the self.* New York: Oxford University Press.
Anderson, L. M., et al. (2003). Culturally competent healthcare systems. *American Journal of Preventive Medicine, 24*(3), 68–79.
Audi, R. (2006). *The Cambridge Dictionary of Philosophy.* New York: Cambridge University Press.
Bryant, J. (1969). *Health and the developing world.* Ithaca: Cornell University Press.
Bynum, W. F., & Porter, R. (2013). *Companion encyclopedia of the history of medicine.* London: Routledge.
Chang, E. S., Simon, M., & Dong, X. (2012). Integrating cultural humility into health care professional education and training. *Advances in Health Sciences Education, 17*(2), 269–278.
Charmaz, K. (1999). Stories of suffering: Subjective tales and research narratives. *Qualitative Health Research, 9*(3), 362–382.
Charon, R. (2001). Narrative medicine: A model for empathy, reflection, profession, and trust. *JAMA, 286*(15), 1897–1902.
Cueto, M. (2004). The origins of primary health care and selective primary health care. *American Journal of Public Health, 94*(11), 1864–1874.
Das, J., Hammer, J., & Leonard, K. (2008). The quality of medical advice in low-income countries. *The Journal of Economic Perspectives, 22*(2), 93–114.
Descartes, R. (1999). *Discourse on method and other related writings.* New York: Penguin Books (Original work published in 1637).
Engel, G. (1977). The new need for a new medical model: A challenge for biomedicine. *Science, 196*(4286), 130.
Ezzy, D. (2000). Illness narratives: Time, hope and HIV. *Social Science & Medicine, 50*(5), 605–617.
Frank, A. W. (1998). Just listening: Narrative and deep illness. *Families, Systems, & Health, 16*(3), 197.
Gofin, J., & Gofin, R. (2005). Community-oriented primary care and primary health care. *American Journal of Public Health, 95*(5), 757–757.
Greenhalgh, T., & Hurwitz, B. (1999). Why study narrative? *BMJ, 318*(7175), 48–50.
Hensel, W. A., Smith, D. D., Barry, D. R., & Foreman, R. (1996). Changes in medical education: the community perspective. *Academic Medicine, 71*(5), 441–446.
Hewa, S., & Hetherington, R. (1995). Specialists without spirit: Limitations of the mechanistic biomedical model. *Theoretical Medicine, 16*.
Institute of Medicine. (1997). *Primary care: America's health in a New Era.* Washington DC: National Academy Press.
Kleinman, A., & Kleinman, J. (1996). The appeal of experience; the dismay of images: Cultural appropriations of suffering in our times. *Daedalus, 125*, 1–23.

Lopez, E., Eng, E., Robinson, N., & Wang, C. (2005). Photovoice as a community-based participatory research method. In B. Israel, E. Eng, A. Schulz, & E. Parker (Eds.), *Methods in community-based participatory research for health* (pp. 326–348). San Francisco: Jossey-Bass.

Mahler, W. T. (1975, May 15). *WHO's mission revisited: Report for 1974 to the 28th World Health Assembly*. WHO Library, Geneva.

McKeown, T. (1976). *The modern rise of population*. New York: Academic Press.

Merleau-Ponty, M. (2012). *Phenomenology of perception* (Donald A. Landes, Trans.). New York: Routledge (Original work published in 1945).

Metzl, J. M., & Hansen, H. (2014). Structural competency: Theorizing a new medical engagement with stigma and inequality. *Social Science & Medicine, 103*, 126–133.

Miller, S. (2009). Cultural humility is the first step to becoming global care providers. *Journal of Obstetric, Gynecologic, & Neonatal Nursing, 38*(1), 92–93.

Muldoon, L. K., Hogg, W. E., & Levitt, M. (2006). Primary care (PC) and primary health care (PHC): What is the difference? *Canadian Journal of Public Health, 7*, 409–411.

Murphy, J. W. (2015). Philosophy, community-based interventions and epidemiology. *Socialinių Mokslų Studijos, 7*(1), 46–59.

Murphy, J. W., & Rigg, K. K. (2014). Clarifying the philosophy behind the community mental health act and community-based interventions. *Journal of Community Psychology, 42*(3), 285–298.

Newell, K. W. (1975). Health care development as an agent of change. In Health in Community Development: International Health Conference: Papers of the Conference on the Dynamics of Change in Health Care and Disease Prevention, October 20-22, 1975, National Council for International Health (p. 5). National Academies.

Newman, S. D. (2010). Evidence-based advocacy: Using photovoice to identify barriers and facilitators to community participation after spinal cord injury. *Rehabilitation Nursing, 35*(2), 47–59.

Paterson, G. (1998). The CMC story, 1968–1998. *Contact, 161*, 3–18.

Paul, D., Ewen, S. C., & Jones, R. (2014). Cultural competence in medical education: aligning the formal, informal and hidden curricula. *Advances in Health Sciences Education, 19*(5), 751–758.

Remen, R. N. (2002). *Kitchen table wisdom: Stories that heal*. New York: Riverhead Books, Pan Australia.

Rifkin, S. B., & Walt, G. (1986). Why health improves: Defining the issues concerning 'comprehensive primary health care' and 'selective primary health care'. *Social Science & Medicine, 23*(6), 559–566.

Rifkin, S. B., Muller, F., & Bichmann, W. (1988). Primary health care: On measuring participation. *Social Science & Medicine, 26*(9), 931–940.

Rigg, K., & Murphy, J. (2013). Storylines as a neglected tool for mental health service providers and researchers. *International Journal of Mental Health & Addiction, 11*(4), 431–440.

Rigg, K. K., Cook, H. H., & Murphy, J. W. (2014). Expanding the scope and relevance of health interventions: Moving beyond clinical trials and behavior change models. *International Journal of Qualitative Studies on Health and Well-Being, 9*, 24743.

Starfield, B. (1994). Is primary care essential? *The Lancet, 344*(8930), 1129–1133.

Stonington, S., & Ratanakul, P. (2014). Is there a global bioethics? End of life in Thailand and the case for local difference. In W. Teays, J. Gordon, & A. Renteln (Eds.), *Global bioethics and human rights: Contemporary issues*. Lanham: Rowman & Littlefield.

Strasser, R., Worley, P., Cristobal, F., Marsh, D. C., Berry, S., Strasser, S., & Ellaway, R. (2015). Putting communities in the driver's seat: The realities of community-engaged medical education. *Academic Medicine, 90*(11), 1466–1470.

Tangwa, R. (2010). *Element of African bioethics in a Western frame*. Mankon, Cameroon: Langaa Research & Publishing Common Initiative Group.

Taylor, C. E. (1976). *Doctors for the villages: Study of rural internships in seven Indian medical colleges*. New York: Asia Publishing House.

Tervalon, M., & Murray-Garcia, J. (1998). Cultural humility versus cultural competence: A critical distinction in defining physician training outcomes in multicultural education. *Journal of Health Care for the Poor and Underserved, 9*(2), 117–125.

Tollman, S. (1991). Community oriented primary care: Origins, evolution, applications. *Social Science & Medicine, 32*(6), 633–642.

True, G., Rigg, K. K., & Butler, A. (2014). Understanding barriers to mental health care for recent war veterans through photovoice. *Qualitative Health Research, 25*, 1443–1455. doi: 10.1177/1049732314562894.

Tsai, J. (2016). *The problem with cultural competency in medical education*. Retrieved from http://www.kevinmd.com/blog/2016/03/problem-cultural-competency-medical-education.html

Unger, J. P., & Killingsworth, J. R. (1986). Selective primary health care: a critical review of methods and results. *Social Science Medicine, 22*(10), 1001–1013.

UNICEF & World Health Organization. (1978). *Primary health care: A joint report*. Alma-Ata, USSR.

Van Lerberghe, W. (2008). *The world health report 2008: Primary health care: Now more than ever*. Geneva: World Health Organization.

Wang, C. C., & Burris, M. (1997). Photovoice: Concept, methodology, and use for participatory needs assessment. *Health Education & Behavior, 24*, 369–387.

Wang, C. C., Yi, W. K., Tao, Z. W., & Carovano, K. (1998). Photovoice as a participatory health promotion strategy. *Health Promotion International, 13*(1), 75–86.

Wang, C. C., Cash, J. L., & Powers, L. S. (2000). Who knows the streets as well as the homeless? Promoting personal and community action through photovoice. *Health Promotion Practice, 1*, 81–89.

Williams, G. (1984). The genesis of chronic illness: Narrative re-construction. *Sociology of Health & Illness, 6*(2), 175–200.

Chapter 10
Conclusion: Reimagining Community Planning in Health Care

Steven L. Arxer and John W. Murphy

Introduction

The idea that health initiatives should be local is not altogether new. Going back to the passage of the Community Mental Health Act of 1963, efforts have been made to decentralize health services so that programs reflect the needs and perspectives of the intended communities. Clearly, a wide range of health practitioners recognize the value of a community's perspective in shaping health care, especially if the intention is for programs to be sustainable in the long run. A central theme of this book, however, is that carrying the moniker of "community based" is not sufficient to ensure that health and other social interventions are relevant to those who utilize these programs. Similarly, projects run from within communities may have established elaborate networks with community members, but these connections may be superficial and short lived. At the core of these problems is the lack of a philosophy to help actualize community-based work. Without a proper guiding theory, projects will run the risk of missing the practices vital to providing community-based health care.

As the chapters in this book have shown, a shift to a new philosophy includes a rethinking of various dimensions of health care, such as epistemology, methodology, leadership, community relations, and politics. Key to all these elements is that community members should be at the center of the planning of social interventions—in this regard, communities sustain program initiatives and determine a

S.L. Arxer (✉)
Department of Sociology & Psychology, University of North Texas at Dallas, Dallas, TX, USA
e-mail: steven.arxer@untdallas.edu

J.W. Murphy
Department of Sociology, University of Miami, Coral Gables, FL, USA
e-mail: j.murphy@miami.edu

project's life cycle. In short, a radical decentering suggests that communities are situated at the center of all aspects of successful interventions. This level of community participation means that social planning is community-defined and community-directed. In line with Beck's (1997, p. 157) notion of "sub-politics," communities control the decision-making process related to their own health and are not obscured by traditional models that privilege the views of experts and other professionals.

Indeed, some of these changes may appear irregular to many readers, but imagining new ways to conceptualize, design, and evaluate projects is part of a community-based approach. A community-based orientation suggests a break, or "de-linking" (Amin 1990), from the conventional realism that has been part of health management. From this new perspective, all aspects of a project are dispersed and can take multiple directions, since interventions are guided by a community's needs and daily social practices (Rochefort 1984). The context of community member participation sets the stage for how protocols, diagnoses, and treatments are developed.

A rejection of dualism is at the heart of a community-based philosophy. Implied by this charge is that the traditional gap between practitioners and communities is misguided. Communities, in short, are not empirical objects and should not be managed and treated from a distance. The reason for this change is simple: communities represent the *praxis* of community members who define and give meaning to their lives. In this regard, what constitutes a community often includes a myriad of perspectives and practices that may go beyond the scope of experts' views. Furthermore, ignoring the constructed character of social life undermines the intentions behind a community-based approach, since the ways in which citizens make their worlds are marginalized or ignored altogether. Health practitioners should thus consider how communities are "embodied" and engage in the hard work that goes along with entering the social world created by these persons (Zaner 1964).

Subsequent to the breakdown of dualism, practically every facet of health services should be rethought. Without dualism to anchor the nature of knowledge and social order, the planning of social interventions should emerge from the bottom-up and reflect the cultural domain of community participants. The locus of these proposals should be based on the history and biographies of the community, so that treatments and other services are attuned to local conditions. A recurring theme in this book is that a realistic portrayal of the world leads to the marginalization of communities since participation is restricted to those who claim objective viewpoints. Nevertheless, ignoring the interpretive character of social life results in programs guided by abstract facts. Community-based projects, therefore, can benefit from a reappraisal of the role of social theory and how a new philosophy can improve the prospects of community planning.

A New Worldview

A recurring theme throughout the chapters of this book has been the important role of participation in community-based work. Highlighting the importance of citizen involvement in projects is to a certain extent almost a cliché. Participation is recognized as a core feature of community-based planning (Leung et al. 2004), and the expectation is to involve community members in every part of a project. For some, engaging the community in this way improves the effectiveness of programs, since local knowledge is gathered and used to sustain research and delivery efforts (McTaggert 1991). While a popular notion is some circles, the distinct philosophical stance being taken may go unnoticed, as well as the profound implications of a participatory model. Most notably, the idea that social interventions should be directed by the indigenous definitions and expectations of a community stands in opposition to the Western intellectual tradition of dualism. Basing health projects in a community represents an epistemological departure from the dualism that has traditionally separated objectivity from participation (Murphy 2014). As a result, community-based philosophy changes the way knowledge production is understood. This shift clears the way for a new strategy that considers the criteria for an appropriate intervention to emanate from local sources.

Community-based philosophy addresses a crucial issue regarding the status of facts. Are facts objective or are they contextual and interpretive? The Western tradition, at least since Descartes, has been clear to privilege objective knowledge divorced from human influences (Bordo 1987). In view of this dualism, opinion is associated with the limits imposed by human perception, while truth transcends these contingencies. Descartes, therefore, believed that to perceive reality clearly, persons must abandon their passions and other idiosyncrasies, so that unbiased knowledge can be gathered. In this regard, Bordo (1987, p. 17) writes that "Cartesianism is nothing if not a passion for separation, purification, and demarcation." Subjectivity and the associated interpretation are a liability that can undermine the collection of factual knowledge.

The denouement of this dualism is that facts should not be considered connected to human action. As a result, factual information has been tied to the "basic rule of the empiricist schools that all knowledge has to prove itself through the *sense certainty* of systematic observation ..." (Habermas 1971, p. 74). Hence facts have been equated with stimuli, sense impressions, and other discrete data. This maneuver intends to ensure that these data are removed from the deleterious consequences of a humanly constructed context. In other words, once facts can escape uncontaminated from cognition, then their applicability is not hindered. A good mind, therefore, acts like a camera and copies the empirical nature of reality. In the end, empirical facts are treated as real and autonomous.

Subjectivity, on the other hand, is considered to be a poor source of true knowledge. For all that emerges from this source are biased interpretations that taint information. Subjectivity represents a fountain of error and must be purged from the knowledge acquisition process, or the related interpretation will obscure the facts. The idea is that impersonal information contains truth, while subjective matters are fallible. Thus becoming objective requires the abandonment of all personal predilections (Straus 1980, p. 119). Any opinions, personal insights, and emotions are invalid unless they can be corroborated by empirical data.

At this juncture, readers should recognize that a community-based perspective abandons dualism. The rationale for this maneuver is linked to the pervasiveness of participation, in that human interpretation and perspective cannot be overcome. What is important is that a pristine knowledge source is untenable, because a clear distinction between human action and the world cannot be sustained. As Lyotard (1984, p. 10) notes, consciousness is not simply a surrogate for reality but rather intimately intertwined with this phenomenon. What he means is that perceptual acts defile and shape whatever is seen, thereby undermining the dualistic worldview. This move away from dualism is often characterized as the "linguistic turn." In this case, the rationale behind the failure of dualism is that the influence of interpretation cannot be avoided, no matter what strategy is employed for this purpose.

A community-based philosophy revels in local definitions and considerations, since they signal how the world is interpreted and organized by a community. Beyond a basic call to include the citizenry, the world is imagined anew. Persons are not simply called to be part of social initiatives but shape these endeavors. From a community-based perspective, personal and collective experiences sustain reality, along with the norms that should guide all interventions. According to Rorty (1991, p. 8), "there is no way to stand outside of all human needs and observe that some of them … are gratified by detecting 'objective sameness and differences in nature'." Social reality is thus never encountered; instead, only particular interpretations are available. How illness is constructed by community members is the focus of a community-based perspective, since local knowledge defines the boundaries that are navigated when becoming sick or seeking treatment.

Community Participation in Planning

Subsequent to the breakdown of dualism, human involvement cannot be divorced from the pursuit of knowledge. The scientific method, for instance, is meant to guide researchers so that their biases and values do not obscure facts (Starr 1982). By following step-by-step guidelines, human perception is constrained and the world is allowed to appear unfettered. However, to borrow from Bourdieu and Wacquant (1992), the relational character of knowledge cannot be escaped. In other words, persons cannot extricate themselves, their values, and perspectives, from the knowledge acquisition process. A perspective from "nowhere" (Nagel 1986) is not possible since human interpretations are pervasive.

Nevertheless, traditional social planning has been predicated on dualistic philosophy. Most notably, experts have been viewed as the best sources of information since they are thought to follow value-free decision-making. Through the use of scientific and technical protocols, experts are said to accumulate untainted facts and possess an unprejudiced view. In this way, social planning is concrete and well founded, otherwise known as "evidence-based" practice (Brownson 2011). In this context, the empirical features of a community, such as demographic characteristics, become the focus. Because these data are easily observable, an accurate portrayal of a community is thought to emerge. Moreover, decisions about community needs are made using statistical models that correlate various empirical indicators to identify social problems. Through what Jacques Ellul (1964) referred to as "technē"—that is, computers and mathematical models—unbiased and thus reliable information is thought to be generated.

Focusing on participation, however, is antagonistic to this approach to planning. Conventionally, widespread inclusion is presumed to invite error in the form of human judgements that occlude a clear view of affairs. More specifically, professionals would need to compete with others when describing community needs and presenting a rationale for an intervention. The claim is that because everyday persons do not necessarily have technical training, they will seriously compromise this process. Despite these concerns, planners who want to be community based must acknowledge that perspectives on knowledge have changed. As phenomenologists might say, access to a pristine world has been eclipsed by a concern for "human interests" (Habermas 1971).

The conventional strategies used to eliminate human bias from knowing and intervening in the world are passé. Without dualism as a starting point, a framework for an intervention must be embodied or situated in a community. Information used for the purposes of planning should thus be recognized as tied to social context, communication, and politics. Issues related to health, for example, are embedded in a complex array of competing experiences and claims.

What this approach suggests is that planning efforts should reflect the everyday ways citizens come to define health and illness and how these realities are part of the symbolic construction of community life. In this way, community-based planning is anchored not in abstract social indicators of a community but rather dialogue and engagement (Scott 1989). For example, as was mentioned in several chapters, advocates of narrative medicine argue that local story lines are the key to successful medical decision-making. Communicative competence, as opposed to technical expertise, paves the way to understanding the facts and issues that are important to a community and warrant attention.

Reimagining Community

Given the interpretive character of social factors, traditional depictions of communities and community relations must be reconsidered. An overly positivistic portrayal of communities has been dominant. Consistent with the Western dualistic tradition, communities have been described in empirical ways, such as systems or bodies. Additionally, in the literature, an ecological model has been adopted that understands community as a matrix of factors, including geographic and demographic features (Poland et al. 2000). Community health, in this case, is the result of how numerous variables (e.g., poverty, age, gender, and education) contribute to health outcomes. An ecological model, nonetheless, presents communities in structural terms that may lead to new forms of reductionism and marginalization.

Such a structural viewpoint ignores how a community is constructed by the interpretive work of its members. Moreover, this conscious activity supplies the meaning that informs individual and community behavior. To borrow from Husserl (1970), empirical indicators fail to capture the "lifeworld" of community members who employ meaning to chart their personal and collective trajectories (Murphy 2012). Poverty, for example, does not causally determine risk behavior. Whether persons identify and respond to a crisis may be tied to how they interpret their futures. In a context of deprivation, persons might imagine a limited future and few long-term benefits to an intervention. This outlook, however, can change with a shift in consciousness. Viewing community to be the product of causal factors is reductionistic because this modus operandi obscures how social life is interpersonally constructed (Bourdieu and Wacquant 1992, p. 96).

Abstract descriptions of a community also marginalize persons from the vital process of community planning. For example, Murphy (2014) notes that the overuse of scientific and empirical descriptions can begin to devalue the meanings community members use to make sense of their everyday lives. Borrowing from the philosophy of Alfred Schutz (1962), he draws attention to how the "primary concepts" used by everyday persons are slowly eclipsed by the "secondary concepts" imposed by professionals to explain behavior. The adoption of the language of variables and causality, for instance, is thought to offer a more concrete representation of community behavior and predictable outcomes. In this way, planning fails to be truly inclusive, since only experts use the proper descriptives.

However, the distinction between technical and everyday language is misplaced. The notions of variables and causality that are used in traditional data modeling are rethought from a community-based perspective. Specifically, a community is not a fixed set of characteristics nor is community behavior reducible to a sequence of variables that produce an effect. This portrayal masks the values and symbolic commitments that are the fabric of community life. Simply put, before a cause can be thought to lead to effect, these two factors must be experientially related. A variable must have meaning to persons that is significantly related to the existence of another variable. This meaning, however, resides only within the history and biography of community, which is a symbolic realm, rather than some empirical association.

Imagining the Communal in Community Action

In light of this new imagery, community action is imagined to be fundamentally a communal affair. While this charge appears to be obvious, the presumed value of community action is not necessarily forthcoming from dualism. Simply stated, a penchant for objectivity and empiricism can lead to normative prescriptions and behavioral expectations that community members confront, as opposed to control. Conventional approaches to community mapping, for example, involve identifying a range of social relationships, resources, and information to develop a holistic portrayal of a locale and chart the best course for an intervention (Corbett and Lydon 2014). Here researchers include community members as sources of input, but directives for planning are tied to empirical features and externalized.

When community action is recognized this way, individuals are assumed to be the passive recipients of the picture painted by experts. How best to design an intervention is tied to descriptives, such as "intensity, frequency, direction, setting, validity, and evidence" (Foss and Rothenberg 1987, p. 254). As a result, persons are entrapped within a framework that they cannot control or direct. The implication is that human action is ancillary to more objective causes of behavior.

This portrayal is unacceptable in a community-based perspective, because behavioral norms are not natural and traceable to an empirical origin. Abstract features, such as location, resources, networks, or community mores, are sustained by a "pragmatic motive," whereby conscious action transforms "natural things into cultural objects" (Schutz and Luckman 1973, p. 5). True community-based mapping, in fact, reveals the stories that are at the heart of this transformation. Hence rather than natural in origin, community order is envisioned to emerge through human interaction.

As a result of the challenge posed by a community-based philosophy, the normative guidelines that shape planning are understood to be situated or tied closely to assumptions that are locally specified. The idea is that community-based interventions cannot be divorced from the experiential contingencies that delimit the rules for normalcy. In this sense, the issue is no longer whether a particular plan is more accurate than another; instead, the goal is to respect the ways in which members establish the identity and parameters of their community's culture. Furthermore, community-based planners are thus expected to encourage this constructive process.

The result is that community-based planners help build a community's world. This coproduced activity entails being sensitive to the process whereby a community weaves together personal and collective narratives to create a sense of community. Here again, a community-based perspective abandons a view that sees a community as simply a collection of characteristics. More than a mere association of traits and individuals, a community is an exercise of *praxis*, whereby various interpretations are established to anchor memories, histories, and identities. As Lyotard describes (1984, pp. 11–14), a community can be found at the intersection of "language games" that are stabilized over time. Community action, in this sense, should be understood as a heterogeneous activity, as persons work to construct and integrate various "lifeworlds." Promoting community action is thus tied to recognizing the communal basis of existence and promoting the interpretive activity that undergirds social life.

Conclusion

A central message throughout this book has been that community-based work is tied to a philosophical outlook. In particular, the dualism that has been associated with conventional portrayals of knowledge, research, service delivery, and community life has significant limitations. Given the focus on participation among community-based advocates and the growing popularity of this outlook among health-care workers, many of the ways in which community planning has been imagined traditionally are outmoded. Appreciating this need to change the basic assumptions that guide health care planning can help practitioners frame their efforts.

While at first a focus on philosophy may appear too abstract for the "on-the-ground" nature of community interventions, projects can benefit from rethinking certain fundamentals. In this case, a rejection of dualism can alleviate many of the epistemological and methodological constraints once thought to be necessary for an effective and successful project. Without being hampered by the restrictions imposed by neutrality and the accompanying objectivity, researchers and practitioners are now free to explore the wealth of information available in communities. As De Hoyos (1989) notes, a realistic view of community occludes the multiple interpretations of reality that are possible. In this way, new dimensions and practices are made visible once the formulaic prescriptions of empirical science are viewed as one among many interpretations of community life. Recognizing the many interactions and interpretations that constitute a community can bring new insights and help promote relevant interventions. But in order for participation to be taken seriously by health care practitioners and planners, an appreciation of this new philosophy that supports community-based work is crucial.

References

Amin, S. (1990). *De-linking: Toward a polycentric world*. London: Zed Books.
Beck, U. (1997). *The reinvention of politics: Rethinking modernity in the global social order*. Cambridge: Polity.
Bordo, S. R. (1987). *The flight of objectivity*. Albany: SUNNY Press.
Bourdieu, P., & Wacquant, L. J. D. (1992). *An invitation to reflexive sociology*. Chicago: University of Chicago.
Brownson, R. C. (2011). *Evidence-based public health*. Oxford: Oxford University Press.
Corbett, J., & Lydon, M. (2014). Community-based mapping: A tool for transformation. In T. Dawson, C. Etmanski, & B. L. Hall (Eds.), *Learning and teaching community-based research: Linking pedagogy to practice* (pp. 113–134). Toronto: University of Toronto Press.
De Hoyos, G. (1989). Person-in-environment: A tri-level practice model. *Social Casework, 70*(3), 131–138.
Ellul, J. (1964). *The technological society*. New York: Random House.
Foss, L., & Rothenberg, K. (1987). *The second medical revolution: From biomedicine to infomedicine*. Boston: Shambhala.
Habermas, J. (1971). *Knowledge and human interests*. Boston: Beacon Press.

Husserl, E. (1970). *The crisis of European science and transcendental phenomenology.* EvanstonIll: Northwestern University Press.

Leung, M. W., Yen, I. H., & Minkler, M. (2004). Community-based participatory research: A promising approach for increasing epidemiology's relevance in the 21st century. *International Journal of Epidemiology, 33*(3), 499–506.

Lyotard, J.-F. (1984). *The postmodern condition: A report on knowledge.* Minneapolis: University of Minnesota Press.

McTaggert, R. (1991). Principles of participatory action research. *Adult Education Quarterly, 41*(3), 168–187.

Murphy, J. W. (2012). *Contemporary social theory: Key themes and analysis.* New York: Springer.

Murphy, J. W. (2014). *Community-based interventions: Philosophy and action.* New York: Springer.

Nagel, T. (1986). *The view from nowhere.* New York: Oxford University Press.

Poland, B., Green, L., & Rootman, I. (2000). *Settings for health promotion: Linking theory and practice.* Thousand Oaks: Sage Publications.

Rochefort, D. A. (1984). Origins of the "third psychiatric revolution": The community mental health centers act of 1963. *Journal of Health Politics, Policy, and Law, 9*(1), 1–30.

Rorty, R. (1991). *Objectivity, relativism, and truth.* Cambridge: University Press.

Schutz, A. (1962). *Collected papers.* The Hague: Nijhoff.

Schutz, A., & Luckmann, T. (1973). *The structure of the life-world.* Evanston: Northwestern University Press.

Scott, D. (1989). Meaning construction and social work practice. *Social Service Review, 63*(1), 39–51.

Starr, P. (1982). *The social transformation of American medicine.* New York: Basic Books.

Straus, E. (1980). *Phenomenological psychology.* New York: Garland Publishing.

Zaner, R. M. (1964). *The problem of embodiment.* The Hague: Nijhoff.

Index

A
Abstracted empiricism, 31
Abstract knowledge, 68
Alma-Ata declaration, 79, 105, 108
American medical education, 96
American medical schools, 97, 102
Anti-dualistic framework, 82, 84
Assembly line medical practice, 61
Associational life, 72
Autonomy, 42

B
Biographical medicine, 17
Biomedical model, 55, 56
    clinical and medical settings, 4, 5
    dualism, 4, 109
Biomedical science research, 31, 81
Biopsychosocial strategy, 15

C
Campbell University School of Osteopathic Medicine (CUSOM), 100
Cartesian dualism, 27
Cartesianism, 16, 121
Centers for Disease Control and Prevention (CDC), 6
Christian Medical Commission (CMC), 107
Commodification of health, 61, 62
Communicative competence, 71, 123
Community action, 124, 125
Community advisory boards (CAB)
    defined, 39
    global health committee, 39
    HAB, 40
    HIV/AIDS vaccines, 39
    local organizations, 38
Community-based approach
    cost of medical care, 1
    health delivery, 26
    quantitative and biomedical, 26
    scientific investigations, 25
Community-based health programs
    "a people's science", 9
    CDC, 6
    defined, 7
    ecological approach, 9
    evolution, 5
Community-based intervention, 65
Community-based leadership, 73
Community-based medical education (CBME)
    American medical schools, 97
    background, 94
    comprehensive assessment, 101
    defined, 95
    hidden curriculum, 94
    osteopathic medical schools, 101
    student-preceptor partnership, 95
    systematic review, 96
    web-based study, 98
    WHO, 94
Community-based participatory research (CBPR), 40

Community-based philosophy, 82–84, 121, 122, 125
Community-based planning, 38, 41, 42, 123
Community-based principles, 38
Community-based work, 119, 121, 126
Community-mapping
  counter-mapping, 89
  democratic and inclusive, 87
  GIS, 86
  identity, 88
  large-scale mapping, 88
  lived experiences, 86
  local residents, 87
  participatory mapping, 87
  perceived distance, 86
  PLA, 88
  spatial clustering, 85
Community Mental Health Act, 18, 119
Community-university integration, 99, 100
Counter-mapping, 89
Credibility of community
  hierarchy and status, 68
  status biases, 69
Cultural competence, 113, 114
Cultural humility, 114
Cultural invasion, 55
Cybernetic hierarchy, 59

D
Dalhousie Health Mentors Program, 96
Decentralization, 73
Deep assumptions, 3
Deficit thinking, 69
Democratization of culture, 74
Democratizing health projects
  community-based leadership, 73
  dialogical knowledge production, 72
  egalitarian spaces, 73, 74
Dialogical knowledge production, 72
Dialogue, 19, 20, 41, 62–64, 83, 88
Distorted communication, 74
Double contingency, 59
Dualism, 4, 16, 27, 30, 57, 60, 82, 109, 120

E
Ecological model, 8, 124
Edward Via College of Osteopathic Medicine (VCOM), 99
Egalitarian Spaces, 73, 74
Emergent coordination, 11
Empirical indictors, 85
Empowerment, 84, 85

Epidemiological studies, 80
Epistemic participation, 31
"Evidence-based" practice, 123
Explanatory models, 21

F
Free-market theory, 60
Full participation, 42

G
Geographic information system (GIS), 86

H
Health advisory board (HABs), 37, 38
  affiliation, 46, 49, 50
  agenda setting, 47, 48
  committee membership, 44
  diversity of projects, 46
  frequency of meetings, 49
  governance structure, 44, 47
  language of advisory, 50
  meeting frequency, 45
  membership, 48, 49
  project, 50
Health-care movement, 79
Health committees
  HAB, 38
  training curricula, 38
  train-the-trainer model, 38
Health promotion model, 1, 3, 5, 9, 79
Healthy urban planning, 80
Hermeneutical injustice, 72
Holism, 21
Holistic medicine, 1, 5, 6, 10
Holistic models, 81

I
Individualism, 60
Interpretive community, 30, 32, 33, 63

L
Language of science, 71
Lifeworld, 30, 31, 71
Lived experiences, 82, 83
Local knowledge, 41, 84
Local ways of knowing
  lived experience, 70, 71
  popular knowledge, 71
Local worlds, 19

Index

M
Medical education, 113
Meetings, 64
Metanarratives, 7
Mind-body connection, 16
Moral pluralism, 111
Mutually satisfying decisions, 72

N
Narrative competence, 17
Narrative medicine, 112
   community participation, 83
   defined, 15, 16
   dialogue, 21
   dualism, 17, 22
   illness domains, 21
   local biographies, 21
   nonrepresentational philosophy, 17
   self-interrogation, 20
Neoliberalism, 61
Normative guidelines, 125

O
Objectification, 4, 82
OpenNotes, 18
Osteopathic medical schools, 101
OurNotes, 18
Over-socialized, 8

P
Participatory action research, 30, 33, 84, 85
Participatory competence, 84
Participatory learning and action (PLA), 88
Participatory mapping, 87
Participatory planning, 85
Patient-centered care, 42, 61
Patient Protection and Affordable Care Act (ACA), 2
People's science, 8, 9, 26
Photovoice, 113
Political community, 56
Positivism, 71
Poverty penalty, 56
Primary care (PC), 106
Primary health care (PHC)
   antidotes, 106
   community-based philosophy, 108, 109
   definition, 105
   narratives, 112
   PC, 106
   phenomenology, 110–112
   photovoice, 113
   vertical model, 107
Pristine social facts, 58

Q
Qualitative methodologies, 26, 82
Quantitative research, 10

R
Reflexivity, 20, 67, 74
Reimagining Community, 123
Research questions and methods, 43
Rural medical services, 107

S
Scientific method, 58, 122
Social constructionism, 74
Social interventions, 119
Social planning, 123
Social reality, 122
Social research, 25
   assumptions, 27
   cartesian dualism, 27
   characteristics, 28
   data gathering, 30
   diagnoses and treatments, 29
   distortion, 28
   dualism, 28, 30
   epistemic participation, 31
   false dualism, 32
   individual and organization health care, 29
   lifeworld, 30, 31
   quantitative techniques, 29
   risk ratios, 28
   social reality, 30
   standardization, 32
   validity, 32
   variable analysis, 32
Sociological analyses, 112
Structural competency, 114
Subjectivism, 65, 82, 121

T
Tak Province Community Ethics Advisory Board, 39
Testimonial injustice, 69
Total market, 60
Train-the-trainer models, 38

U
University of Maryland School
 of Medicine, 99
University of Washington School of Medicine
 (UW), 100

W
West Virginia University School of Medicine, 99
WHO European Healthy Cities project, 80
World entry, 19, 63, 64
Worldview, 122

GPSR Compliance
The European Union's (EU) General Product Safety Regulation (GPSR) is a set of rules that requires consumer products to be safe and our obligations to ensure this.

If you have any concerns about our products, you can contact us on

ProductSafety@springernature.com

In case Publisher is established outside the EU, the EU authorized representative is:

Springer Nature Customer Service Center GmbH
Europaplatz 3
69115 Heidelberg, Germany

www.ingramcontent.com/pod-product-compliance
Lightning Source LLC
LaVergne TN
LVHW021334080526
838202LV00003B/165